THE PSYCHOSOMATIC THERAPY CASEBOOK

THE PSYCHOSOMATIC THERAPY CASEBOOK
Stories from the Intersection of Mind and Body

Jean Benjamin Stora

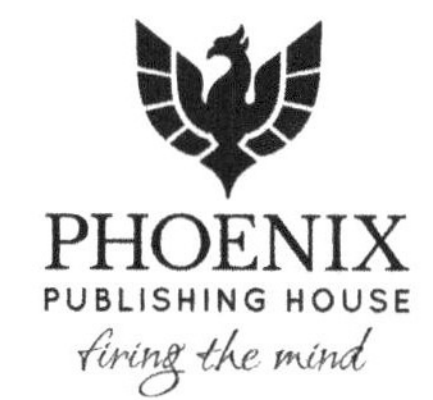

PHOENIX
PUBLISHING HOUSE
firing the mind

Originally published in French in 2019 as *15 cas de thérapies psychosomatiques: Comment soigner les malades, non simplement leurs maladies* by Les éditions Hermann

First published in English in 2023 by
Phoenix Publishing House Ltd
62 Bucknell Road
Bicester
Oxfordshire OX26 2DS

British Library Cataloguing in Publication Data

A C.I.P. for this book is available from the British Library

ISBN-13: 978-1-800131-44-6

Typeset by Medlar Publishing Solutions Pvt Ltd, India

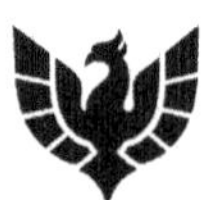

www.firingthemind.com

To my dear wife,
Professor Judith Stora-Sándor

To my dear son,
Michael Stora, psychoanalyst, psychosomatist,
and clinical psychologist

Contents

About the author

Jean Benjamin Stora is the Honorary Dean of the Faculty of the School of Higher Commercial Studies of Paris (HEC) and a practicing psycho-analyst and psychosomatist. His professional practice began in 1973 and his teaching in 1960. He chaired the Institute of Psychosomatics "Pierre Marty" from 1989 to 1992 and the French Society of Psychosomatic Medicine from 2000 to 2002. He created and ran the consultation of Psychosomatics from 1993 to 2015 at the Pitié-Salpêtrière Hospital, and the Diploma of Integrative Psychosomatics, Psychoanalysis, Medicine, and Neurosciences at the Faculty of Medicine of the Pitié-Salpêtrière, UPMC Paris 6 from 2006 to 2015. He is the current Director of the Institute of Integrative Psychosomatics of the Society of Integrative Psychosomatics. Jean Benjamin Stora's work is in the tradition of Melanie Klein, W. R. Bion, and D. W. Winnicott.

A mysterious word: "psychosomatics"

I worked from 1993 to 2015 as a psychosomatist at the Pitié-Salpêtrière Hospital. I created this consultative position, which was first located in the rheumatology department and then in the endocrinology department, thanks to my friendly relationship with Professor Jean-François Allilaire, Head of the Department of Psychiatry. Psychosomatics is neither endocrinology nor rheumatology, being a discipline that deals with the mind in relation to the body; therefore, I was available to the medical services throughout the hospital. Teachers and doctors were aware of the existence of my position, and some of them referred patients to me.

To please the department head and the doctors, I wore the same scrubs as them, with a red badge on which was written: "Psychosomatist". The doctors who saw this badge for the first time opened their eyes wide to understand what it said and who they were dealing with! During those years, I met and investigated nearly 4,500 patients suffering from all types of pathologies. They trusted me and we maintained a very cordial relationship for many years. I cared for them, and this book owes them much, as it does the doctors, my colleagues, with whom I worked and with whom I shared concerns. You will then ask me, "How did you treat them? How did you do it?" The answers to your questions are in this book. But first, remember that psychosomatics concerns all pathologies and that it is not an *imaginary* disease. In my opinion, all diseases are psychosomatic since the human being is a psychosomatic unit.

In the West, doctors treat the body and are trained in medical schools to care for the organs of the body and their functions, which they must fully understand in order to become doctors. They have at their disposal magnificent techniques and extraordinary exploration devices. As one of my colleagues at the Faculty of Medicine, who was a friend, said: "Here, technique dominates the relationship of care." His statement was quite true, as was revealed in my relationship with the physicians in my department to whom I wanted to communicate the results of my observations. They did not listen to me, because they were busy and had too much work, which I always understood.

So, I spent my time developing a patient-observation method so as to communicate it to my university degree students at the Faculty of Medicine. Using this method, I drew up a summary of my observations, which joined the medical reports in the patients' medical files. The only colleagues I could talk to about my observations were, ultimately, the nurses and a hospital practitioner who became a very great friend and with whom I continue a dialogue. My consulting office was not on the nurses' hospital ward—it was in another building—so they welcomed me very warmly into their office, where we were able to talk extensively about the results of my investigations and about my patients. Although I left the hospital several years ago, I maintain a very warm relationship with my former colleagues.

In customary medical practice, the medical examination is not followed by questions about the patient's life or the relationship of this narrative to somatic disorders from infancy onwards. Physicians treat the bodies of patients in the present—in the here and now, as psychoanalysts say. But who are these patients? How did they get sick? Answering these questions would take up too much time and doctors have no training in talking to patients. When investigations lead to dead ends, a diagnosis is impossible: doctors are at the limits of their knowledge and thus often declare that it is a question of a "psychosomatic disorder", by which they mean an *imaginary* disorder of the patient's mind.

It is at this point that I intervene with patients to continue exploring the relationship between the mind—that is to say, psychic functioning—and somatic disorders, real or imaginary. First, I want to tell you that, for me, there is no psychic *causality* of any somatic illness. In the discipline I have developed, the mind, or psychic system, *participates* in all diseases, without being the cause. Thus, when I hear such statements as: "You are the person responsible for your illness," I dismiss any psychic causality. There is nothing more terrible than such a statement because no individual is directly responsible for their illness. It is obvious that many dietary, addictive, and other behaviours can eventually cause an imbalance of homeostasis, leading to somatic disorders. The body has defence systems that allow it to cope for many years, but after ten or fifteen years the imbalances start to become evident. I totally agree with medicine in this regard.

That being so, when I knock on the door of one of the rooms of our service to visit my patients—and not just those presenting with psychiatric disorders—I introduce myself to the patient; as you must know, a "shrink" worries many patients because of false beliefs in mental illnesses. I dispel any misunderstanding by stating that as a psychosomatist, and with their help, I am going to explore their current and past life history in relation to all the somatic disorders they have had in their lifetime. Once the relationship of trust is established at the patient's bedside, it is possible to have very long interviews: forty-five minutes, one hour, or more. Patients disclose, talk about their often-difficult lives, and, for the first time, find "someone to talk to about themselves". You are going to ask me what I do with their story? As you will read in this book, I use a method that allows me to better understand and evaluate the relationship between the mind, or psychic functioning, and the somatic disorders for which the patient has come to consult me. I can then offer them therapeutic support, a psychosomatic therapy, or immediate help to get them through the difficulties they are experiencing. These proposals are complementary to the medical treatment they are receiving and do not, in any way, contradict the prescriptions of my colleagues.

In order to better understand the new approach that I call "integrative psychosomatics", this book presents the therapeutic progress in the cases of fifteen patients, and of other patients I have treated in the last twenty years: of Georges suffering from hyperlipidaemia, and Gilles, Ariane, Elvire, Emma, etc. You will, thus, better understand the therapeutic method that is complementary to the medical approach. In integrative psychosomatics, it is necessary to perform two roles in order to treat patients: that of a psychosomatist therapist and that of a doctor.

This is always a bit more complicated than it appears, and it is important to understand that the central nervous system is fundamental in the relationship between mind and body. Therefore, to complete this holistic approach, I appeal to neuroscience. You will see with Emma, who is a brain-damaged patient, how we can modify the therapeutic method to address the brain of the patient thanks to the knowledge of neuroscience; a new discipline has emerged, namely neuropsychoanalysis.

In integrative psychosomatics, the basic hypothesis is that we are confronted every day with excitations of varying degrees. Alongside the immune system, the mind—or psychic system—is a second line of defence against these excitations, gradually enabling them to disperse so that they do not disrupt our lives. This can create intense stress on a daily basis. The working of the mind, like that of the immune system, can thus be significantly disrupted, making it unable to handle excitations. These are transmitted to the central nervous system, which then has the task of managing them. The excitations follow different neural circuits, activating, for example, the autonomic nervous system, but also the immune system as well as other somatic systems. It is understandable, then, that excitations should be treated at the level of functions and of somatic organs with their own systems of defence. When excitations persist (e.g. traumatic events, grief, etc.), the homeostasis of organs and functions is disrupted and somatic disorders appear. This book will describe numerous dysfunctions of the mind or psychic system and the appearance of somatic disorders.

Treating the body without healing the mind may, eventually, cause the movement of disorders from one disease to another. To the great surprise of doctors, one disease can replace another—that is, the one they healed.

The first four chapters of this book present fifteen clinical cases—so fifteen stories—and these can be read by the majority of patients (and general readers); the fifth and final chapter is specifically intended for therapists and doctors wishing to understand the practice of psychosomatic therapies, the technical points of which are reviewed in this chapter. However, patients can also benefit from reading this last chapter, as well as the conclusion, which will enable them to understand the difference between psychoanalytic technique and the technique of psychosomatic therapy.

As part of this introduction, I would like to warmly thank my colleagues—professors from the Faculty of Medicine who participated in the university degree courses I created, as well as the doctors from my endocrinology department; and finally, and especially, all the patients and patients who trusted me. I have walked with them all these years.

CHAPTER 1

Doctors, patients, and mind therapists

The human being is a psychosomatic unit

Some preliminary questions need to be asked before the themes of this chapter are addressed.

The doctor and his relationship with the patient

What do we learn about the doctor at the Faculty of Medicine? What are the goals that the doctor pursues in order treat and cure? In the usual allopathic medical approach, how does the doctor evaluate the risk of diseases, the risk of medical practice in his daily exercise?

The question is: where is the patient? In privileging the body, is the "mind", and especially the story, of the patient not forgotten? Do doctors know their patients? We talk about the body of the patient: but which body? What is the nature of the doctor–patient relationship? And what about the mind of the doctor? What is the quality of life? Does the doctor cure diseases, treat sick people? What are the expectations of the doctor? The patient must follow the prescriptions of the doctor: what happens to patients who do not observe them?

The patient and his body

What is the patient aware of in relation to the disease? What does he search for, unconsciously and consciously? What are his expectations of the doctor? The problems of the relations of the mind and the body of patients are complex: the fears, the feeling of getting better, how to interpret the signals sent by the body.

Psychosomatist, patient, and doctor

Complex and potentially conflicting relationships exist in attempting to understand the mind in its relation to the body: can the mind make one sick? Does the body have an influence on the mind? How can the unity of body and mind be restored? In the same way that the body can deny disease, can the mind oppose the healing of the body? Can the body disrupt the functioning of the mind? How can a psychosomatist, a sick person, and a doctor work together to heal? Is it possible to heal?

These are some of the questions that integrative psychosomatics proposes to answer.

To care for the body and the mind, to care for the mind in its relation to the body and to care for the body in its relation to the mind constitutes a scientific and therapeutic challenge that has not yet been solved in France. The approach of psychosomatic doctor Professor Bonfils, the doctors of Saint-Antoine, Montpellier, Toulouse, Bordeaux, as well as the approaches of the psychoanalytical psychosomatic schools of Pierre Marty and Sami Ali, have failed to convince the faculties of medicine to introduce the psychic dimension of somatic patients into their curricula, just as psychosomatic psychoanalytic schools have not succeeded in developing an approach to the physical problems, the bodily disorders, of patients. We continue to focus only on the "psyche" body and not on the real body affected by the disease. Psychoanalysts ignore the diseases of the bodies of their patients; the same is true of allopathic doctors, who are unaware of the life events of their patients. The best we can expect is that, at least, the mind is valued by psychiatry!

This non-recognition of the relationship of body and mind can be found in current statistics: 85 per cent of doctors do not have their own doctor! They treat themselves and prescribe medication when they are ill. How does one explain this lack of confidence and this inability to trust in medicine? The professional stress of doctors is very high, and it is only recently that we have started to worry about it. Doctors are human beings like the patients they care for. "No one is safe from somatisations," as Joyce McDougall (1989) said.

The same is true of the efficacy of allopathic medicine, which can be seen in the epidemiological statistics of treatment adherence: very often, at the end of a year, more than 50 per cent of patients no longer follow to their treatment! What then is the effectiveness of medicine if patients no longer take their medication? Young doctors in the faculties and in their hospital placements have no training in relation to the patient. They stick to technical considerations of biological analysis or very brief records of patients' antecedents, something to which I have been witness for twenty-one years at the Pitié-Salpêtrière. Recently—and we must, at least, recognise this progress—therapeutic education and patient information have appeared, and we want to salute these first steps. But is it enough just to listen to and understand patients? These approaches are very focused on knowledge and behaviour. There is total ignorance of the functioning of the human unconscious and the processes of a psychic thought.

How to treat the patients rather than the disease

How can patients be treated when the doctor takes only a few minutes to make a diagnosis and prescribe medication? What does the doctor know about his patient's life? How can the life events of the patient, and their effects on health, be considered in the diagnosis?

For twenty-one years (from 1993 to 2015) I practiced as a psychosomatic consultant at the Pitié-Salpêtrière Hospital, consulting both patients in my department and those from other departments: cardiology, urology, nephrology, neurology, diabetology, etc. I will begin by talking about Georges.

Georges: the integrative psychosomatic approach

Georges will help us better understand the professional practices of doctors and therapists. As his case progresses I will make comments, as a psychosomatist, integrating the approach of medicine and the approach of the new model of psychic functioning developed for somatic patients. (In Chapter Five, I will present the meta-psychological reference model of integrative psychosomatic psychology.)

Georges was referred to me by my colleagues in the endocrinology department four years ago. He has Type IV hyperlipidaemia with a very low level of HDL cholesterol, which is an indication of possible prognosis of myocardial infarction. He also suffers from hypertriglyceridemia. It began in the May of the previous a year, with back pain in the left shoulder blade; the patient called a doctor and was hospitalised urgently for myocardial infarction. He was hospitalised for twenty days for post-infarction rehabilitation. The surgeons inserted a 3mm by 20mm Wiktor stent; they also confirmed kidney failure. Georges, who was then thirty-three years old, had stopped practicing sport more than twelve years previously. His fifty-six-year-old father is overweight, he is also a big smoker; his mother, fifty-five, is overweight and suffers from phlebitis. Georges is a tall man—more than 1.85 meters—and at the time of his infarction weighed 103 kilograms.

That is as much as my medical colleagues told me, because that is how they examine all our patients. Based on symptoms, they make a diagnosis (based on epidemiological studies) and a prognosis and prescribe hospital procedures and medication.

We can ask ourselves questions. Do the doctors know Georges? Who is Georges? Is it necessary to know him, especially when one is facing an influx of patients? George suffers from a chronic illness, and if we want to treat him in the long term and prevent any cardiovascular risk, it is imperative to know who George is beyond the biological parameters.

A female doctor, who was sensitive to the personal dimension of patients, referred Georges to me for psychosomatic examination. This interview will open the door on the exploration of George's "psyche" and his life. As we proceed, I will indicate what this can bring to the patient's understanding and to the improvement of the care that can be provided.

At the time of the interview Georges is thirty-five years old. I spent more than an hour with him: a very nice man, with a depressive tendency, whose responses shifted between the seductive attentions of myself and one of my interns and our questions about his inner state and his anxieties about the future. When I meet him for the first time, he presents a smiling face in anticipation of the interview, and his behaviour reflects a demand for immediate attention and trust.

First thoughts: meeting a "psychiatrist" at the hospital

Patients are always worried about meeting a "shrink"; somatic patients are not mentally ill, and our first duty is to reassure them about their psychic integrity. Georges' seductive behaviour is of the child–mother type, as in the first relationships. Georges asks to be accepted and to receive affection. I answer all these requests with a smile that reflects his smile. I am like a caring and empathic mirror. I recommend to my students that in the first minutes of a meeting they create an unconscious space in which to welcome and receive the patient and his words. The patient will know immediately that he is understood and no longer just heard; he feels accepted and that a relationship of trust can be established without even knowing the people he meets because they are caring and empathetic.

Continuation of the interview

He begins to tell me about his heart attack in May following intense work stress. He works as a salesman in a computer company and waiting for results and short-term goals has placed him under unbearable pressure; occasionally he criticises the society in which we live, while accepting its restrictions.

Reflections

Why does Georges so stoically accept such a situation? This is the question I silently ask myself and to which he will provide an answer. His speech, in which parental authority emerges, which expresses a tacit acceptance of professional constraint, reflects the relationship with a father who has been authoritarian throughout the years of childhood and adolescence. He talks little about his father and mother (as if they did not exist), but a lot about his grandfather, a Central European Slav, and his Mediterranean grandmother, with whom he grew up. His grandfather, in loyalty to his host country, adopted the language and culture of France so that Georges did not learn to speak the language of his ancestors, but it seemed to me during our interview that he sounded his "t"s as the Slavs generally do when they speak French.

He seems deeply in search of his identity with his nostalgic expression of a return to the family home to end his days (why does death appear?) far from the problems of the city. He sounds like a hermit when he talks about retiring to this house built into the mountain, accessible by a narrow path that will one day be transformed into a track for cars. He wants to retire in six to ten years after putting his money into a few houses that will bring in enough for him to survive. Retire at forty-five? What is going on?

The professional stress has deeply affected Georges, who dreams of a return to the family home in the next ten years while he is still very young. Depression appears very clearly in this fantasy of refuge and everyday disillusion. We can note several traits of character in the first minutes of our interview: first, the severity of paternal authority, the extreme requirement to achieve lofty goals, namely, an ego ideal set up from earliest childhood; then the romantic nostalgia for the house of the grandparents, close to his heart, the imaginary place where he can take refuge; then a spiritual dimension, encouraged by an uncle which he speaks about with me later in the context of his psychotherapeutic treatment, an uncle with whom he identifies. Georges lives in permanent conflict (between tyrannical ego and superego) that forces him to relieve all his tensions in his work. Georges is the victim of an ego ideal that considerably limits his ability to find solutions in his professional life and in his life in general.

What is striking and poignant in someone so young is to feel inhabited, several times during the interview, by death. He looks back on his adolescence and his passion for women. He married young, at the age of eighteen, and quickly had two children. Because of his early marriage, Georges had to give up long-term study; he had been dating a young girl with whom he had fallen in love, and as she was expecting a child, her parents forced her to marry. Throughout his therapy, Georges spoke in a romantic and nostalgic way about his first wife with whom he had two children, boys he continues to care for. The death presents in his speech is metaphorical in nature; and involves a major falling away of drive energy, of vitality.

It is towards the end of the interview that he recognises that it was the pressure of his family environment that forced him to marry a young woman he had got pregnant. His love life had until then been very short, and he was suddenly promoted to being the head of a family; he knew he had not been mature and wondered if he had still not achieved it! Throughout the interview, he initially presented a version of his marriage as if it had been a passionate affair, only to finally recognise that this passion was being lived with another young woman whom he had met three years after his marriage. This young woman belonged to a religion different from his own; his passion for Sabrina was intense and still continues, since this evocation brings him to tears and he suddenly understands that it is not forgotten and that he has not drawn a definitive line under this episode in his life. In fact, this passion led him to divorce; his wife has since remarried and he deeply regrets not having stayed with here, nor to have maintained a connection, but, again, he was immature, he did not understand anything about life. He had let himself be carried away by his passion for women. He never dared to introduce his children to Sabrina as he did not want his two children to have a bad opinion of their father.

Psychosomatist's comment (anamnesis and therapeutic strategy)

The first questions that arise are first: what is the defence capacity of the patient's psychic functioning system? What are the points of fixation and regression in the psychosexual maturation? Is the maternal object introjected?

Clinical experience tells us that somatic patients who fixed in archaic and pre-genital positions in their developments are more fragile than patients fixed in phallic and genital positions. I refer to the meta-psychological model developed by Sigmund Freud that has been modified for somatic patients by reintroducing intrauterine phases and the first years or archaic phases of development. All these stages were established by eminent doctors and psychoanalysts: Dr Rene Arpad Spitz, Melanie Klein, Donald Winnicott, Wilfred Bion, Daniel Stern, etc.

During this investigation, we can advance the hypothesis of a double fixation: in the crucial period when the oedipal organisation should have been developed but was not; and in an oral fixation which determined the feeding behaviour of the patient, leading to the cardiovascular risks he has faced. In the therapeutic relationship, we are clearly aware of the immaturity of the patient as well as a fixation on the mother of the first stages of life and on the mother of adolescence: nostalgia and romanticism create a love that he cannot give up (we are here in the presence of one of the first phases of the unresolved oedipal conflict), a romantic love to which he has remained fixed and which determines the choice of his love relationships.

I must mention here the mourning for the first love (his wife he left when he was twenty-one years old), then the mourning for the second love, which is not yet done with and which the patient continues to suffer. We are therefore in the presence of two bereavements and of a depressive symptomatology that forced the patient to offload all his energy into the work; there is no other opportunity to discharge tension since Georges no longer practices sport. For each patient it is important to evaluate what Freud calls the economic dimension, namely the investment of libidinal energy and, I will add, somatic energy in several activities and in general human relations. Due to a grandiose self-ideal,[1] Georges is limited in the investment capacities of his mental and somatic energy. This limitation led him to a very great depletion that favoured myocardial infarction. The mental defences being insufficient to manage the number of daily excitations, these were transmitted, via the central nervous system, to the sympathetic and parasympathetic

---

[1] For Heinz Kohut, the balance of primary narcissism is disturbed by the inevitable gaps in maternal care, but the child restores initial perfection by establishing a grandiose and exhibitionist image of the self (the grandiose self) and by abandoning the previous perfection to an admired and omnipotent transitional self-object: the idealised parental image. The term "grandiose self" (Kohut, 1971) is used to describe the structure based on fantasies of grandeur and exhibitionism that is the counterpart of the idealised parental image.

nervous system. Ultimately it is the heart organ that absorbs the excitations, until it eventually gives way.

I present at the end of the chapter a diagram of psychosomatic investigation that I have drawn up to facilitate the initial investigations and the establishment of a diagnosis, and you will find below a list of all the theoretical and clinical questions that a psychosomatist puts to a patient.

Theoretical and clinical questions of the psychosomatist

---

1. Relationship to the mother in the first years of life:
   - Has the object been introjected? The relation to the maternal object has, above all, been developed by Melanie Klein; the mother of the first stages of life will be progressively internalised after nine months. The strength of the early-life connection allows for the development of secure effective relationships in later life and the pursuit of life in a balanced way. We therefore understand the importance of asking the question about the presence of a maternal object.
   - Maternal deficiency or maternal depression during pregnancy, after the birth of the child, in the first year of life, or in the first five to six years of life, etc.
   - Relationship with the mother in the first six years of life and formation of character traits and behaviours. The investigative therapeutic relation must make it possible to establish: absence of the object (dead mother, deficiency, depression, etc.) opening the way to somatisations; fusion with the object (the child has never detached from the mother of origin); cleavage of the object, good mother/bad mother; attachment to the pre-object (the approach of Melanie Klein); introjected object (internalised), facilitating the process of development of the psychic system, deeply connected to the immune system.
   - relationship to the father in childhood and adolescence.
   - Mental representations of the parental couple.
2. Basic problems of psychic identity and cultural, autobiographical self-constitution:
   - Development of identity in the family, the lived identity (various manifestations during the history of the subject), problems of the development of sexual psychic identity (childhood and adolescence, especially repression of sexuality).

- Influence of the cultural environment on psychic development; this dimension is often ignored by therapists in France (ignorance of Judaism, Islam, Chinese culture, Japanese culture, etc.).

3. Psychic assessment of antecedents:
   - Level of anxiety related to the age of onset of family members' illness (father, mother, grandparents, brothers, sisters, etc.).
   - Age of death of parents in relation to the age of the patient. In some cases, the patient imagines that they cannot go beyond the parents' age of death, as if they have reached the limit of their life!

4. Evaluation of the imaginary life, or as Pierre Marty says, the thickness of the preconscious:
   - Cultural beliefs that are symbolised without mental representations.
   - Beliefs with mental representations.
   - Evaluation of associative capacities: the existence of associative chains with the present–past round trip; representations of things and representations of words.
   - School life, high school, university: memories, evaluate community channels.
   - Evaluation of the imagination during critical periods of life: childhood, adolescence, first dating, social life, professional life, career development.

5. Assessing the resources of the patient: how can they economically mobilise energy to survive disease?
   - Imaginary life and cultural and sporting leisure. Reading? Music? Theatre? Cinema? Television? Internet? Attendance at clubs or cultural groups?
   - Social, artistic, sports, etc.
   - Political and union activities.
   - Spiritual beliefs: whatever the belief, it is important to know that it can enable the human being to survive.
   - Nocturnal dreaming and daydreaming.
   - How are life projects developed? Do they follow the patterns suggested by parental education? (Here, psychic expression of the ego and the superego or the ideal of the ego.)

6. Trauma:
   - Childhood, adolescence, adulthood.
   - In the family: being beaten, violence, etc.

- In professional life: professional stress, harassment, "burn out", etc.
- Accidents, divorce, dismissal, etc.
- Socio-economic, political, etc.
- Physical environment: earthquakes, etc.

7. Repetition mechanism
   - To connect with the identification mechanism to the father and the mother in the first years of life, then in adolescence.
   - To relate to the experience of identity in the family environment.
   - Repetition of maternal destiny.
   - Repetition of paternal destiny.
   - Choice of the partner on the manner of identification to the father and the mother.
   - Choice of the partner as an external object (substitution object).
   - Repetition of psychic distance from the object by substituting it for geographical distance (allergic object relation).
   - Repetition of the choice of the object on the manner of the aggressor object (masochistic type relationship).
   - Repetition on the narcissistic mode: choice of the narcissistic object in a mirror, or choice of the object according to the ideal of the self (father or mother or environment).

8. Usual operating modes:
   - Sexual impulses: the significance of seduction in the relationship with the psychosomatist in respect of the infantile manner of searching for maternal love, or a multiplicity of states of seduction until the genital stage. It is important to note the narcissistic dimension to assess the nature of the seduction. The person tries to seduce in order to seek the love of the object or to feed his or her narcissism, to look in the mirror of the other.
   - Aggressive impulses (self-aggressive and destructive impulses).

9. Drive fusion and drive defusion, drive defusion and diseases, reversal of aggressive impulses against self, self-destruction:
   The search for an aggressor by somatic patients implies a drive defusion that inhibits the projection outside aggressive impulses that continue to destroy the human being. At best, the sexual drives and aggressive impulses of a human being are interrelated. When this is not the case, aggressive impulses can turn against a human being in manifestations of self-destruction and can fuel the disease.

10. Fixation points and addictions as indicative signs of early deficiencies, sensorimotor fixations:

    Fixation points are indicative of stopping the development of psychosexual maturation of the development of human beings. Many life events can then be origins of these fixations that will eventually determine traits of character, behaviour, and investment of energy resources in different vital activities.

    - Narcissistic dimension.
    - Masochistic dimension.

11. Diseases—economic dimension:

    - Never forget that the disease reaches the libidinal economy of the psychosomatic unit. The disease absorbs somatic energy and libidinal energy.
    - The disease (somatic function or organ) absorbs libidinal energy, so any loss of libido is to be assessed according to the severity of the somatic diseases.
    - Evaluate the investment capacity by the life impulses of projects, the pursuit of active life, relational capacities, investment of leisure activities, etc.
    - How does the patient use his or her psychic energy?
    - Importance of metabolic energy available to the patient.

Continuing theoretical and clinical reflection on Georges

Georges is a religious man, developing, between Roman Catholicism and Orthodox Catholicism, something that seems closer to what he feels inside. He is a very sensitive spiritually oriented being who takes refuge in the church to regain inner calm, near God. He left Sabrina, and I feel that this is to punish himself for having broken his bonds with his wife, for not having been faithful to paternal guidance and that of God!

He hates the company in which he has worked up until now: in truth, because of the forced marriage (it is me that states this), he could not study and started work at a young age. He earns a good living and is very proud of it. He met a third woman who looked after him during his heart attack, and from whom he separated a year later because she wanted to marry him, have children, etc. Unlike in his relationship with Sabrina, he introduced her to his children. Confronted again with a choice that reactivated his multiple experiences of love and pain, Georges made an extreme decision depriving himself of emotional support. Georges is alone, his apartment is not yet furnished, he lives in the middle of his cardboard boxes and other packages.

Depression is watching; she is present in all aspects of Georges' life. He has been a great sportsman, but he is currently suffering from myalgia, a side effects of his medication for cholesterol. High levels of cholesterol may have contributed to the formation of atheromatous plaques eventually reaching the coronaries. Georges eating habits are very bad for his health, and he has not made any changes to these. Although it is necessary, he still hasn't started any sporting activities. This young man went through a depressive phase before the heart attack and following it and the separation from his companion, etc.

At his place of work, his role has been changed: he has a more sedentary job, but the work is as intense and, like all executives, he leaves work very late.

Psychosomatic therapy

We will see at the end of this book the psychosomatic nosography to establish a diagnosis, but for George, given the infarction and depression, it was strongly recommended that he go into treatment.

I therefore saw Georges once a week at the hospital for more than three years. From the first sessions, I was confronted with the omnipotence of his narcissism. The most difficult aspect has been the integration of the narcissistic stream[2] into the entire process of psychosexual maturation and into what is called the genital tract. This is a necessary step that had never been integrated.

Georges is a man aware of his power; he acts as if he feels invulnerable; he deliberately ignores his body of which he demands considerable effort. A predominantly narcissistic being is unaware of living in a body. He is animated by a vital current that lends him his qualities of

---

[2] The narcissism of the first stages of life must, through a well-conducted education, gradually integrate into what is called the genital tract. This process is necessary so that the ego can gradually become autonomous and take psychic control of the different functions of the psychosexual process.

omnipotence, invulnerability, and sometimes the eradication of time and space (see Grunberger, 2003). He works more than twelve hours a day and goes home completely exhausted, to feed on extremely lipid meals. He lives in an apartment he has not fitted out, and his current depression is of no help in unpacking all the cardboard boxed that clutter up the rooms.

Georges is a great seducer and has no problem appealing to the many women who are attracted to him. There is a repetition mechanism at work in all his relations with women: Georges projects onto the woman he as met the image of the ideal woman he dreams of, a "pure" woman, to whom he swears to devote his life. After a few days, a few weeks, or a few months, Georges leaves the young woman because she does not correspond to his ideal representation. We must understand that this ideal image can refer to the mother of his adolescence endowed with all the attributes of seduction (an archaic and oedipal conflict). This is an ideal image that can never be found in reality.

He has another fixed idea, inspired by his grandparents' house where he spent his early childhood. He dreams of restoring the house and settling there when he turns 40 and retires. This is once again a grandiose dream about the future. What characterises Georges is the omnipotence of the grandiose self (Kohut, 1971) which distances him from reality and keeps him in an unreal universe.

The psychotherapeutic strategy consists of gradually inserting the principle of reality into the patient's narcissistic and instinctual universe. It took a long time before Georges allowed himself to join the world of everyday reality. After three years of psychotherapy, he is thinking of leaving his job to retrain professionally so that he can live his life differently and change the pace of his life.

The psychodynamic and economic changes achieved makes it possible to better regulate the patient's eating behaviour; results are also obtained thanks to the resumption of sports practice. The progressive integration of narcissism into the genital drive tract allows the process of psychosexual maturation to resume and ensure the patient's homeostasis over time. Georges has resumed his life in a different way; he is actively involved in his professional redeployment, has finally bought an apartment which he has fitted out so as to live there comfortably, and he plans to restore the family home to spend holidays there with his children, rather than to go there to die. During his therapy, his understanding of his relationship with his father and his mother was considerably deepened and the oedipal conflict began to be addressed.

The process of maturation is on track, and Georges' health has improved.

The integration of narcissism makes it possible to place at the disposal of the patient's personality large quantities of energy that he can use to better direct his life in the real world. The analysis of the conflicts with the superego and the ego ideal make it possible to gradually strengthen the capacity of autonomy in daily decision-making. The patient can, for the first time, attend to the reorientation of his professional life and his life. The psychic system is a very important line of defence, since it links up behaviours, emotions, and mental representations. A well-constituted psychic system must be capable of absorbing a very high quantum of excitations, thus ensuring that these excitations are no transmitted to the various somatic systems. This is not what happens when the psychic system is compromised. Not all patients have an apparatus built on the model of the classic neurotic described by Sigmund Freud; there are many flaws in the process of maturation because of failures and deficits of the psychic system. It is the same on the genetic level concerning the organs and somatic functions.

When the psychic system is confronted with a very high quantum of excitations that it cannot control, these excitations are transmitted to the somatic functions through neural systems. It was here that the psychosomatic integrative approach originated because psychoanalytically inspired practitioners had been considering only the faults of the psychic system, ignoring the role played by the central nervous system and the autonomic nervous system that relay excitations. The psychoanalytic metapsychology created by Sigmund Freud was never intended to explain somatisations. We find ourselves here at the epistemological limit of psychoanalysis.

The neuroscientific dimension of the body in somatisations

The body expresses its primary response to mental stress through the autonomic system and endocrine activity. Endocrine activity is expressed through the responses of the adrenomedullary sympathetic system, the pituitary and adrenocortical system, and the thyroid. The main hormones of the adrenomedullary sympathetic response are epinephrine and norepinephrine. Mental stress induces a heterogeneous response of catecholamines. Differential activation occurs at different sites of the sympathetic nervous system. The main hormones in the pituitary and adrenocortical responses are adrenocorticotrophin and cortisol. All research in the field of mental stress (see Stora, 2007) and the cardiovascular system carried out to date shows that mental stress triggers responses of the cardiovascular system as well as cardiac disorders. Although, the exact nature and extent of the causes of cardiovascular disease are still unclear, uncontrollable mental stress is understood to have the ability to induce cardiovascular responses in humans.

The hypothesis that I put forward in the case of Georges, as well as in the cases of the myocardial infarction of many patients, concerns the effect of *permanent* mental stress and not of *acute* mental stress. Although it is difficult to prove that permanent mental stress induces cardiovascular disease, many researchers believe that mental stress is one of the multiple factors causing cardiac ischemia and arrhythmia; permanent stress is also among the risk factors for cardiovascular disease, including hypertension. This argument is difficult to resolve because we do not have objective methods to quantify levels of chronic mental stress. What we can consider, in a multifactorial model of the disease, are the different psychological characteristics present in heart disease.

Mourning a close relative is stress that can increase the risk of heart death. The studies by Merz, Krantz, and Rosinski (1993) and Reich (1983) show that the mental stress induced by the death of a partner causes a 40 per cent increase in the mortality rate of men during the first six months following the death of the partner, two thirds of these deaths being due to a cardiovascular disease. Impaired Type-A personalities have competitive behaviours, ambition accompanied by aggressive manifestations, and are likely to develop cardiovascular disease. The indications are that the correlation is very weak; however, recent research establishes that the Type-A behaviour is of men and women of action who have difficulty controlling and regulating their behaviour (as in Georges' case). These are the subjects who are at high risk of cardiovascular disease.

In a twenty-year longitudinal study (the Framingham Study), Eaker, Abbott, and Kannell demonstrate that Type-A subjects have twice as high a risk of angina pectoris than Type-B subjects. Another eight-and-a-half-year study (Rosenman et al., 1976), with a large cohort of Type-A and Type-B subjects found that Type-A patients had more coronary disorders than Type-B subjects. Anxiety and depression are predictors of heart problems in patients with coronary heart disease. Research reveals very strong correlations between the state of chronic anxiety, depression, and the states of angina and sudden death. Friedman et al. (1986) demonstrate that the phenomenon of depression that develops during myocardial infarction continues during the post-infarction period. We can understand here that if it is not accompanied by supportive psychotherapeutic treatments the depressive state can only aggravate the health of the patient in the post-infarction period. (Here, we can better understand my decision to engage Georges in a psychosomatic therapy.)

Studies undertaken in the 1950s about the formation of atheroma plaques, and, therefore, atherogenesis, tell us that in the period of intense stress preceding income tax returns, accountants have very high cholesterol levels compared to those reported at other times of the year. Significant research suggests that the aroused state of the central nervous system is accompanied by activation of the pituitary-medial medullary-sympathetic system or activation of the pituitary-adrenocortical system; both systems help to increase lipaemia and ultimately atherosclerosis. Glucocorticoids and catecholamines both facilitate the release of fatty acids from adipose tissue, and cortisol directly stimulates hepatic production of very low-density lipoproteins. The increased release of free fatty acids may be inhibited by propranolol, suggesting a beta-adrenergic mechanism.

Studies in the field of mental stress and sudden cardiac death (SDC, or Takotsubo or broken-heart syndrome) tell us that mental stress can cause heart problems, lower the threshold of ventricular fibrillation, and cause cardiac arrhythmias, especially when there is coronary heart disease. Such mechanisms are at work in sudden cardiac death. Development of coronary heart disease, the degree of left-ventricular dysfunction, and the presence of cardiac arrhythmias determine the patient's vulnerability to mental stress causing sudden cardiac death.

Mental stressors contributing to sudden cardiac death include grief, unemployment, social status, level of education, degree of mental stress, social isolation, and disruptions to the life of an individual. Approximately 20 per cent of patients with ventricular arrhythmias may have causes of mental stress. The mechanisms of the sympathetic system and the parasympathetic system contribute to sudden cardiac death induced by mental stress; other factors are the influence of myocardial injury on ventricular innervation, myocardial sensitivity to arrhythmias, thyroxine, glucocorticoids, insulin, and the status of the central nervous system. The increase in sympathetic neuronal activity predisposes a person to dysrhythmias. In summary, many of the studies found that permanent stress was associated with very high levels of cholesterol.

Primary prevention of coronary heart disease should include the reduction of mental stress in the family, at the workplace, and in the community. Secondary prevention should include behaviour modification, treatment of depression and anxiety that cause post-myocardial disorders, prevention of social isolation, and reduction of global stress.

Gilles: the relationship between the somatic body and the disease

Gilles is a sixty-five-year-old man. He has had diabetes for twenty-five years. His current hospitalisation is due to an infection located in the big toe of the right foot, and probably about to spread to the neighbouring toe. The question of amputation arises.

With regard to the medical file: Gilles has had glaucoma since the age of twenty-five; he was diagnosed with viral meningitis at the age of thirty-two; he has "hepatitis B" indicated as "long-standing"; gastroenteritis (in the part of the stomach just before the pylorus); bilateral hypoacusis; Dupuytren's contracture; arterial angiopathy of the left leg; and several surgeries: sympathectomy, varicose vein surgery on the left leg; an operation on the Dupuytren's contracture; and an amputation of the toes of the left foot. He has serious heart problems. This is a multi-medical, polysomatic patient, and there is a question of very great fragility of the mental defences during the last forty years. Anamnesis should provide more information in this regard. I hypothesise a continuous overflow of the psychic apparatus by daily excitations being regularly and rapidly transmitted to the level of the somatic systems that absorb them by affecting their homeostasis. We must also understand that each level of a living being has its system of defences and that the body goes to a second level when the first no longer ensures homeostasis.

At the time of my first meeting with Gilles, the medical decision about amputation has not yet made; the question is whether to amputate or to consider other attempts at disinfection. Gilles willingly agrees to a discussion with me, which I interpret as a positive sign for our continuing relationship. At the outset he announces that he is "anxious", "depressed", that he "wants to cry". It is perhaps these words, but also the rather acute tone of his voice and his sad and pleading expression, that make me think of a child, a child who needs to be pitied and calmed down. Why does he want to cry? He feels alone. He is used to hospitals, however: before his retirement, he worked in this very hospital as a nursing assistant.

A phone call interrupts the beginning of this interview. To the person on the other end of the line (who was, I learned, his daughter), Gilles announces that a psychologist has come to visit him. I hear him say: "Because I may need it." After hanging up, Gilles tells me that it was his daughter, his adopted daughter Khadidja, whom he adopted at the age of four months and who is now twenty-four. Khadidja's biological parents had wanted to abandon her; Gilles managed to place her in the hospital nursery. Regarding the adoption, there was a whole judicial process, and Gilles "fought like a lion" because Khadidja's parents opposed her adoption. He succeeded in getting full adoption rights, which he does not regret at all. His daughter calls him several times a day: to say hello, to ask how he has eaten, and to say goodnight to him. She's "a good girl".

To my question of whether he is married, Gilles says he "stopped all that" in order not to "traumatise" his daughter! How should these words be interpreted? Why deprive Khadija of a maternal presence!

Khadidja is of Kabyle origin. She is very beautiful; this is something that is often remarked upon to Gilles. She chooses her own friends. She had wanted to become a psychologist, but Gilles explained that was just an idea—"nothing at all". She then trained as an educator. "She has a very hard character. She has a strong need to exercise authority."

I mentally note that his daughter is very present beside Gilles, but I also think of the fact that he feels alone; I then bring up his "depression" and the anguish he told me about at the beginning of the interview.

Gilles then talks about the rehabilitation centre where he stayed after his amputation. Because the centre was outside Paris, his daughter could not visit him. What especially "depressed" Gilles were "all those disabled" young people without arms or legs, who "laugh all the time", which seemed to him incredible. "What can I complain about?", he said several times. In silence, I think about his upcoming amputation, which he did not seem to relate to his experience with young people with disabilities. When we talk about his diabetes, Gilles says straight away: "It's mum who had diabetes." His mother had had one leg amputated. There were thirteen children in the family, of whom only two sisters and one brother are still alive. Several of the siblings had diabetes, but Gilles took a complicated blood test (it took several days) thanks to which he knows that there is no genetic element in his diabetes. "I don't care whether there's a family factor or not, anyway the disease is there," he adds.

Gilles relates that during one of his hospitalisations he was "sent" a psychologist because—he thinks—of what he said to a nurse: "I'm fed up, I want to finish with all this." (Gilles laughs, seeming to be very satisfied with the anxiety this caused the nurse.) "But no," he said, "I would never have done that": it would be at odds with his religion, it is only God who can decide to take life back. He goes on to say that he is "disappointed with God". "It's because of mother, she was a saint, she had thirteen children and she remained a little bit of a mother-hen." It is also the hospital that is involved in this disappointment. To my question "Because of too much suffering?", Gilles answers, "Not mine, I don't care." Gilles says he is "someone who keeps everything to himself, who doesn't show anything." He mentions hypoglycaemia, expressing the discomfort that one feels in this state. This leads him to express his rancour about the indifference of people: "You can fall in the street and nobody will come to help you; people think you're a drug addict or an alcoholic …" Regarding his experience of finding out about his diabetes, Gilles says that, at first, he was not worried. He had realised that he had diabetes, because his mouth felt dry. But it was only "when the arteries became blocked" that the disease began to worry him.

I remind him that he'd already come across diabetes: it was a disease his mother had. He agrees, yes, and then his brother, his sister … He says he could have had cancer or leukaemia, it's something we don't choose … He says that the rehabilitation centre "completed me". When I ask him to clarify what he means by that, he says he has no right to complain; he has never imagined being disabled, cancers, leukaemia, yes, but "not that". It affected him a lot. Regarding the cause of his current hospitalisation, Gilles says he has a wound in the "finger" of the foot, an infected wound that does not heal. He says he prefers to have this toe cut off, explaining this by the fact that the previous amputation (he makes a gesture in the direction of his mutilated left foot) went very well, that it healed quickly. It's also because the doctors have told him that the infection is "going to the next finger".

Gilles says he wants it to end so he can go to North Africa. He's been holidaying in the same place for the last thirty years. But he does not know if the amputation is going to happen or not. Gilles expresses his dissatisfaction with the attitude of the doctors on this morning's rounds: they spoke to each other as if it wasn't him being talked about, and he wasn't told anything specific; he is looking forward to next Tuesday (today is Friday) when he should be told about the next stage of treatment (whether he will go to the clinic for the amputation or not). Here we can see evidence of the extent of the distance between the hospital doctor and his patient. For more than twenty years I have witnessed this distance, which doctors are not always aware of. No effort is made to enable the patient to understand his condition, nor to reassure him. Doctors talk to each other! I ask about the quality of his sleep and his dreams: is he dreaming? He says he sleeps well, more or less; he has dreams. He dreams from time to time of his family, those who have died. He has nightmares from time to time, but "in general things are fine".

Towards the end of the first interview, Gilles says, in a trembling voice, almost crying, that he would like to have another three to four years to make some trips … He is in a hurry to leave for the Maghreb; seeing his friends is more important to him than seeing his family. He repeats that for a long time he has been to the same place for his holidays. He adds with a smile that his daughter "is fed up", that she does not want to go with him anymore. When I propose to Gilles that for this first meeting we stop there, he agrees and says he will watch television.

He then begins to talk about various facts he has heard on television, asking me if I am aware of this or that fact. He talks about the increase of suicide attempts among adolescents; he then goes on to the case of "paedophile priests", which he speaks about at length, expressing an astonishment mixed with indignation. A few moments of silence follow this monologue, a silence during which I feel that Gilles is waiting for a reaction from me. "It touched you, this story," I say. "Yes," he continues, he finds it incredible: in his day we could never have imagined it. I agree and let a few moments pass, then propose to Gilles that we end the interview and I come back to see him in a few days. He agrees: "Come whenever you want," he tells me.

A few days later, I meet Gilles again: he seems sad to me. Yet Gilles' comments contradict this first impression: he says he's getting better. He tells me about the visits he had this weekend: his daughter and—big surprise!—someone Gilles recently met during his stay at the rehabilitation centre: a young man, a Maghrebin, who had been a patient at the centre. He "doesn't have both arms". He had asked permission from the centre and came to visit Gilles. I suggest we talk about the history of this friendship, and Gilles says that they "sympathised" with each other at the rehabilitation centre, explaining this by the fact that he not only knows this man's country of origin but, in particular, the place where he lives. They had arranged to meet there. Gilles is impatient to go there; he is thinking of leaving towards the end of the month (our meeting is at the beginning of the month).

Mentioning again the "good surprise" of the weekend, Gilles returns to the young man and his disabilty. With astonishment hiding his disapproval, he insists that the young man has many plans: he wants to get married and have children. Gilles expresses his concern about the young man's future wife—she will have to look after him "like a baby"; for example, he must remove his prostheses to take a shower. Gilles' statements remind me of numerous psychological and practical problems that I have encountered with patients with disabilities. These human beings have the right to a life like everyone else, and we must help them in this regard; it seems that Gilles often makes very harsh judgements, which hide anxiety about the loss of his own limbs.

I share my feeling with Gilles that he seems a bit sad today. He brings up his fatigue: he has been lying down for four months. I ask him how his foot is. "It's getting better," he says, his foot is "almost healed". He also talks about his next trip to the clinic (the same place he would go to for the amputation): this time it is "scratching" that is planned. He adds that it would not bother him if "the finger" was cut off. Gilles again mentions his wish to leave for the Maghreb. I remind him that he said that seeing his Maghrebin friends is more important for him than seeing his own family members. "But I do not have a family!" he then says. I say that I had meant the brothers and sisters he had spoken to me about during our last meeting. "We do not see each other," Gilles says. "They are racists," he adds after a pause. He says that when they lived together, Gilles, returning from his vacation in the Maghreb, often brought "someone" with him. This caused discontent in his family. Later, when Gilles lived in his own apartment, his guests could stay for a month, a month and a half (we are gradually seeing the "others", from the Maghreb, as his new family).

This leads Gilles to talking about his current home: it has a balcony, the view is very nice, you can see the whole of Paris. He really likes the neighbourhood, he likes going out, shopping; when he's not too tired, he goes to Chinatown, it's cheaper. But, recently, Chinese shops have started to be "dirty", this is not like before … After a short break, Gilles exclaims: "But they are not dirtier than the Arabs!" I repeat, "Dirty?" Gilles goes on to say that it is not a question of "those who are *there*" but of "those who are *here*". Those who are "there" are "great people", they "are not dirty at all, on the contrary". "Those of us here are different"; Gilles speaks of the difficult conditions of the lives of emigrants in France, bringing his reflection back to the fact that "a young man, he is Arab in his family, and when he goes out, he is French". Gilles does not like Paris. When the sun shines, everything is all right, but when it rains … He was born in Marseille; his parents had left Italy. He does not know his family in Italy. (We can now better understand Gilles' preferences and his yearning for the southern Mediterranean.)

Following one of my questions, Gilles talks about his Maghrebin friends: he got to know them during a visit. The father was a taxi driver; Gilles has used his services several times, they have "gotten on well", and, little by little, Gilles has "entered the family". Since then, he always goes to their home; they also call each other. Gilles tells the story of his relationship with a young man from Algeria, an English teacher, who was an undocumented immigrant. Gilles had met him several times at the supermarket, they "got on well", they set up several meetings (and the young man always came). Gilles invited him to his home, his daughter found him "nice". At the time, this young man was staying in a hotel with another undocumented immigrant. Gilles suggested that the young man stay with him, which he did for several months. Gilles talks about the benefits of them living together: this young man helped Gilles' daughter with maths, helped her with her studies, brought her to the Centre Pompidou, introduced her to the internet. Algeria is a beautiful country, and it is almost as beautiful as France. Gilles brought his daughter to Algeria to introduce her to her origins. But Algerians are "stupid", they do not know how to use the country's resources. They did not have many specialists; young people leave to study and do not want to return. The situation is very difficult there.

I ask Gilles if Khadidja's parents still live in Algeria. He confirms that they do. Khadidja's mother is "not serious": she had two daughters with the same man (even though they were never married, he says). She remarried and she had two more sons. "She's not serious," her daughter says; she does not want to see her mother again. "Well, she's the one who sees …"

The interview is interrupted by a nursing assistant who has brought Gilles some milk. He tells me he does not eat lunch or dinner. To my question about this abstinence, Gilles explains that while on the one hand, it is not good, on the other hand, he does not want to put on weight "There are some, they eat, they drink, they smoke. If I were like that, I'd be done for already," he says. As with the first interview, my proposal to take a break for this meeting is followed by agreement and, immediately afterward, by a monologue from Gilles. He advises me to visit Algeria; we would have to use this or that agency, not take a charter, go there in the spring, etc. As I get up to leave the room, Gilles laughs: "It's me who was the psychologist today."

Seven days later, we meet for the third time: Gilles receives me by announcing that the amputation has been performed: "I've had two fingers removed," he says. "But I made a mistake," he immediately continues: he had got up to go to the bathroom and had fallen. There was blood everywhere; two nurses helped him up; they "shouted" at him, but afterward apologised. "It was a surprise," says Gilles. Not grasping what

Gilles means by "surprise" (the amputation? the fall?), I begin to formulate my question: "You did not expect …" Gilles interrupts me, saying: "Yesterday it was terrible …" I ask Gilles what the problem is exactly. He talks about the drugs he has been given, medication that does not completely calm the pain. "The professor, the head of the department, refused to prescribe morphine," he says. He is taking another drug; he must have "100 mg" but what he's being given is "50 mg" and that is not enough. This medicine "acts on the head", he does not feel "normal", "drugged". That worries him. As if to escape from the present moment, Gilles talks about his friends from the Maghreb: he has phoned them, they know. They told him that they had built a room with a kitchen "at the top" of their house. The father of the family (the former taxi driver) is working at the airport at the moment, but he does not like working there … He tells Gilles that when he comes, they will work out together what they are going to do. His friends are very grateful to Gilles, they often thank him for everything he has done for them.

To my question of what he has done for them, Gilles says, "Not much … gifts … things of value—huh?—jeans etc." He goes on to say that his pension here is not much; in the Maghreb it is different … Gilles returns to the story of the meeting with his friends: the father of the family is a taxi driver, he has left Gilles his phone number, so Gilles calls him when he needs a taxi. Sometimes he has to wait because his friend is racing, so Gilles waits for him. Once, Gilles's daughter went to Algeria with her boyfriend, having been invited by this family; they went to their home, so Gilles and his daughter became "more friendly" with this family. Gilles and his daughter have been going to Algeria since her childhood. They first went to holiday parks; sometimes it was two stars, sometimes three stars, and often, two stars were better than three! During one of these trips, Gilles and his daughter met a family (they were eating at the same table). They "got on", and these people suggested that they return the following year at the same time. Gilles' daughter went there alone. She was not happy with her vacation because Gilles did not give her permission to go beyond the holiday club. He told her that she had enough things to do inside (sailing, swimming …).

His daughter travelled a lot alone. The first time, at the age of four, she had gone to see Gilles' sister in Germany. She did not want to go back there anymore: Gilles' sister is a severe woman, and the education she gives to her children is very different from the one Gilles gave her daughter, who she says is very spoiled. I point out that since we have been talking, he has expressed a strong preference for the countries of North Africa as if they represent a new family for him, a country of adoption. "Yes," confirms Gilles, he likes Algeria a lot. Algeria is more expensive than the other countries of the Maghreb, but he stopped going there because of his daughter. What happened? He wanted to protect his daughter. Once, he and his daughter had gone to Algeria. She was between four and six years old at the time. They were in a hotel. Khadija's parents had threatened to "take her back tomorrow at 11am". So Gilles has booked emergency flights back to France. To do this, he "lied" by saying that his daughter was very sick. Gilles also "lied" to the hotel staff to justify their hasty departure; with a week's stay at the hotel still booked, Gilles had announced his decision to spend the rest of his holidays with friends who had invited him and his daughter. The next morning, Gilles and his daughter took a taxi and returned to France. I ask Gilles to clarify whether Khadidja's parents had the legal power to take her back. No, but he did not want to traumatise her. The meeting with both parents was violent: he fought with them, he had "hit them both"!

At my request to clarify how it happened, Gilles says: "My daughter was in a room with her parents; she was sleeping. The parents were kissing each other; the man held his arm around the shoulders of the woman (Gilles mimes this gesture) while the man touched the little girl's vagina with his finger!" Was this Gilles' fantasy? Gilles said he had seen them; he became angry, he accused the mother of being a "slut", a "whore". Gilles acts out this scene by pointing his index finger and saying angrily: "Towelhead!", "Filthy foreigner!". He also said that he had described this episode to "the judge". "They are all like that, it's like Africans," he told the judge. Gilles says of himself: "That's the Arabs, there it's part of the culture." Listening to this story, one wonders whether it is fantasy, and especially whether there is an unconscious meaning. I ask Gilles if his daughter has any memory of this distant episode. "No," he replies, "she was too small." But she does not want to see her parents anymore.

This episode allows us to return to the story of the adoption of his daughter. The story begins with Gilles' meeting with the brother of Khadidja's future biological father: Gilles helped him out a lot during his stay as a student in France. To thank him, he invited him to Algeria for his holidays. Gilles went and was very well received by his friend's family. Gilles specifies at this point in the story that these events took place well before the adoption. It was during his stay in Algeria that Gilles met the father of the future adopted girl. Later, he came to France with his girlfriend; they were not married, insists Gilles several times. It was during this stay that Khadidja was born. The couple, unable to look after their baby, who at this point was three months old, brought her to Gilles, who had no way of caring for the baby: he was living in the hospital caretaker's room. He had a West Indian friend at this time. Gilles told the couple that he could not take responsibility for the child. Parents had only one solution: to leave the child at the DDASS (the adoption office). For Gilles this was unbearable; he contacted the parents and all three back to the DDASS to get the girl.

I ask Gilles: "What was so unbearable for you?" "The baby's eyes," he says. She looked at him as if she were saying, "Take me, take me, take me …" Later, Khadija's mother wrote Gilles a letter giving him the legal rights of adoption of the child. After going through various stages, he was granted plenary adoption. I think, then, of this strange situation: of a single man adopting a baby! Can Gille manage without there being a mother? I ask Gilles if there was not, at that time, a woman who could have played the role of mother to his adopted daughter. "No," says Gilles, "I did not want that." Moreover, because of his diabetes, he could not "have intercourse …" (What is the reality of Gilles' genital sexuality?)

Given an archaic fixation in the process of psychosexual maturation, Gilles has an infantile personality; he has not become a psychic adult with an oedipal conflict. One can better understand his search for affection. After a moment's silence, I say that this renunciation had been difficult for him. "No," responds Gilles. For him, sex is, above all, "sterile". He has never had a "really strong relationship" with a woman. Consequently, he put everything onto his daughter. He took care of her: she "gave him measles … the diseases of childhood, eh?" Then, it was rhinopharyngitis … But he never regretted it … Gilles settled into a maternal role.

I try to clarify with Gilles the chronology of some events, namely the dates of adoption of her daughter and the onset of his diabetes. He does not remember anymore: "It was more or less the same time …" He comes back once more to the adoption of his daughter and declares that he has never regretted it. She comes to visit him, she brings her dirty laundry … She is very well educated. When she tells someone that she is an adopted child, she is told, "You can congratulate your father." She is happy. "And you too?" I add. "Yes," says Gilles, laughing.

So, we end our final interview because I don't believe I will meet Gilles again as he has to go to the rehabilitation centre; I wish him a good recovery. Gilles thanks me for our meetings!

Therapeutic and medical comments and guidelines

Listening to the patient's unconscious with one's own unconscious is the usual procedure in taking somatic patient history: what can be said after these three anamnestic interview sessions?

First, Gilles' relations with women will reveal to us at what point in his process of development the patient has remained fixed, which will have determined every aspect of his behavioural pattern with women. Gilles told me about his mother, his adopted daughter, the biological mother of his daughter, his Antillean friend, the female judge, calling them mother hens, not serious … in truth women are almost non-existent in his life. He reduces sex to "sterile relationships". I see there a blockage of the sexual drive, which appeared very early by fixing the patient in an archaic phase of development. He has an ideal image of his mother, and, on the level of emotions he has remained psychically a child. This little child cannot assume an objectal adult genital sexuality[3] because he has never reached this stage of development. He is always looking for a maternal relationship, which he finds in the choice of North Africa as a country of origin, and in the search for families who can welcome and take care of it. This is how we can explain his relational system: welcoming people, hosting young Maghrebins, putting up families for more or less limited periods, and maintaining emotional relations in North Africa. If the father is absent in Gilles' speech,

---

[3] Human beings can, up to a certain age, reproduce biologically and have sex. Establishing adult object relations requires that the human being has reached the last stage of psychic development of psychosexual maturity: the genital stage and the Oedipus complex. Otherwise, we are in the presence of people constantly looking for a maternal object as part of their romantic and psycho-affective relationships.

we can hypothesise that, just as in the first relations, father and mother are mingled before being progressively differentiated in the process of maturation.

Illness has been part of Gilles' entire life. Whenever he has been confronted with events that he could not mentalize, the excitations passed to the level of the soma, which responded with its own specific defences. We do not know if the two events—the adoption of his daughter, and diabetes—can be related. Gilles chose to be a nursing assistant as if, by identification with his mother, to fulfil a benevolent maternal role vis-à-vis patients. Knowing that the patients that Gilles cared for had "cancer and leukaemia", the words "I could have had cancer or leukaemia, we do not choose" can be seen to be a reference to the role played by disease in the psychosomatic body. Gilles, by the way, confirms that he had not been aware of the seriousness of the diabetes when he was told about it by the doctors. The fate of his diabetic mother was there in the background, like a threat. The vision of the disabled amputee's members was traumatic, as if it had caused some sort of psychic blindness hiding the amputation of his own mother.

The opposition of "pure" and "dirty" is even more revealing of this archaic fixation; at a certain stage of development, we are in the presence of the paranoid–schizoid nucleus[4] described by Melanie Klein, making it possible to reject what is dirty outside and to keep inside what is pure. Gilles has not reached the stage of ambivalence and understanding of human behaviour. At this stage of human development, the child has not yet established an integrated picture of the relationship with others. We are in a period of cleavage: good and bad, pure and dirty. All that is negative cannot be preserved within the developing psyche; the negative is projected outside the mother whose primary role is to give an explanation that will allow the child to understand the universe in which he lives.

---

[4] The paranoid–schizoid nucleus develops in the first months of life of human beings; we are in the presence of the baby's perception of a good mother and a bad mother. These two images will merge at the age of nine months. Meanwhile all that is unpleasant and unbearable is projected outside by the child onto his mother who must give meaning to what disturbs him. This is an important maternal role, absorbing the unpleasant and giving meaning to the projections of the child as he seeks to get rid of what disturbs him.

The first narcissistic fixation leads to a specific way of thinking about self-generation and the creation of a new family. Gilles created new familial and effective relationships based on the model of dependence that he knows perfectly, and that he has repeated throughout his life. The psychic cleavage has allowed him to establish pseudo-family relations; we can understand his speech being tinged with "xenophobia and racism" if we link this speech to the archaic stage of development at which Gilles is fixed. At this point, all that exists is the good and the bad. A human being fixed at this stage does not understand what racism is, and especially not ambivalence!

Dorothy and Gilles: the relationship of the psychic body to the sick body

Doctors take care of the physical body, and they study for years to learn how it works. But can we stop at the functioning of the organs and various somatic systems? Can we reduce a human being to his body? This question is, in my eyes, central to the psychosomatic approach.

I would first like to present here the story of Dorothy and her doctors (de Viel, 2010):

> Dorothy has been living alone since the death of her husband ten years ago. Despite her intense desire to remain independent and autonomous, she must be admitted to the local hospital to explore her diabetes, which is becoming more and more unstable. A few days later, Dr John ..., psychiatrist, and his wife, who have been her neighbours for many years, go to visit her in the hospital on her ninetieth birthday ... When her good neighbours ask her how she is doing, she hesitates for several seconds. Then in a calm voice: "Good. A very kind young doctor came and examined my ulcers on my old feet; a woman doctor came to see my eyes; then a specialist came to listen to my heart." Feeling that she did not seem totally satisfied with the care despite the explorations, the psychiatrist invited her to say more. Again, she hesitated, sighed, and, staring at her neighbour, replied: "Well, I have a doctor for my feet, one for my eyes, one for my heart, but I don't feel I have a doctor for me." Dorothy's story resembles

> those of my heart or kidney transplant patients who confessed
> to me: "The doctor is very nice, he looks after my transplanted
> heart, my transplanted kidney, but he doesn't take care of me!"

In integrative psychosomatic, the real body possesses an image at the level of the central nervous system to enable it to manage all the somatic functions. The real body is the body familiar to the doctors who learn about it during their years of study. Outside the real body, there is the body that the spirit inhabits. The psychic system develops during the first twenty years of life and establishes relationships with the different somatic systems throughout the psychosexual development of individuals. The psyche gradually invests the organs with its energy, called libidinal energy, which allows a human being to take pleasure during the years of maturation and later in the rest of his life. Without this libidinal energy, the human body is only a robotic biological body. Pleasure accompanies each stage of development. The problem becomes complex when we understand that, in every society, there are many prohibitions relating to the sexual behaviour of individuals, especially in the last stage, namely, the genital stage of development. Prohibitions and repression can completely block the biological and psychic sexual functioning of human beings. The failure to invest psychic energy in the biological organs leads to many somatic disorders, revealing the disarray of human beings in the face of the genital sexual drive.

A human body that is not totally invested by the libido is deprived of access to pleasure, cut off from the neuronal centres of satisfaction; it is a body reduced to an organic functioning limited to a certain number of immune and genetic defences. It is a fragile and vulnerable body, unprotected by psychic defences; a body reduced to quasi-robotic operation, without a soul.

There is, therefore, a second body, a second *image* of the body, which is the "psychic" body. Our patient Gilles has a relationship with the body that reveals that we are situated at the level of the real body, the organic body: the relationship with his diseased legs and his encounters with the disabled people at the rehabilitation centre suggest that Gilles is maintaining considerable distance from the suffering caused by the "castration" of the hands, arms, legs; this is either to put the suffering at arm's length or, especially, not to feel these as attacks on the real body. Nothing exists: not the pleasure of touching, not the pleasure of walking, etc. Gilles can take care of his body only if he is helped by maternal substitutes; he is like a little dependent child. That's why I recommend that in his case he have a weekly relationship with a nurse from the diabetes clinic who can follow him at a distance, to monitor his condition diabetes and his long-term prognosis.[5]

Therapeutic recommendations are at the same time simple and complex as far as Gilles is concerned. He intuitively found new families to receive affection, help, and support if needed. He found surrogate parents. We can only encourage him in this, and, if by chance, he is taken into therapy, the main objective will be the introjection of a maternal object that will allow him a little more autonomy.

Ariane: when the mind invests the body—the vulvodynia of Ariane and the exploration of a medical mystery by integrative psychosomatics

When the vulva, which includes all the external female genitals, becomes painful without medical examination finding the cause, the doctors speak of vulvodynia. As it can last for months or even years, it is very important that it be followed by a doctor who is trusted and who recognises this disease: it is not "in the head" that this is happening, even if this chronic affection ends up affecting morale ... The cause of vulvodynia is not known. This affection is all the more mysterious in that it can occur suddenly, without following a particular event, and last for months or years before disappearing![6]

Among the treatments for vulvodynia, physiotherapy, corticosteroids, and local anaesthetics are used to relieve pain, and, in the most disabling forms, some antidepressants have been shown to be effective.

---

[5] We will see other later cases where I will further develop the problem of the relation to the real body and to the psychic body.

[6] Information from the following sources: the website www.doctissimo.fr (in an article by Dr Jesus Cardenas, updated 6 June 2016); *The Merck Manual of Diagnosis and Therapy* (Paris, 2008); and the website of the French National College of Gynaecologists and Obstetricians, www.cngof.asso.fr

The article quoted in footnote 6 makes no reference to approaches other than a medical approach in the strictest sense. There appears to be total ignorance of the psychosomatic dimension to human beings. Therefore, for the attention of gynaecologists, I will put forward some reflections from a clinical case.

Ariane is in her thirties and has suffered from vulvodynia with vaginismus for about two years; she experiences pain on a daily basis, which initially led her to consult a psychoanalyst. The psychoanalytic treatment had no effect because, in my clinical experience of somatic patients, this case is not appropriate to be dealt with the technique of classical psychoanalysis: this is not a criticism of psychoanalysis; the problem is not of an oedipal nature. As a teenager, Ariane had seen a psychotherapist for two or three years because at puberty she had suffered from somatic disorders—mainly of the intestines—accompanied by anxiety.

One can already wonder about the nature of the disorder and the anal fixation of the patient. We can hypothesise about difficulties of internal control, revealed by the somatic symptom. Very often this type of symptom tells us that sphincter education is still under the control of the mother. The archaic mother failed to allow her child autonomy, and now the child cannot control her body. Ariane is a very talented student who wants to go to university. She goes abroad to study comparative literature but when she returns to France she falls again into depression, which impels her to consult a new therapist. Again, therapy does not work!

Ariane describes her mother as very protective and often sick. As for her father, she states that he is a very severe man, devoid of empathy, not understanding of his daughter at all; for him, his daughter's somatic troubles are unimportant. She decides to leave the parental home, suffering very soon after from repeated attacks of colitis; she then has an operation to treat an anal fistula. In each of the therapy sessions, Ariane describes at length the somatic disorders in the belly, bladder, bowel, and genitals. Ariane has missed her vocation as a doctor, and like many patients whom I have met, she has, a defence, invested intellectually in the field of medicine; she demonstrates her encyclopaedic knowledge about her somatic disorders, rather than relating to them. There is a complete absence of imagination with regard to the psychic investment of her organs and her somatic functioning. About two years before the symptom of vulvodynia, she had undergone surgery for diverticulum of the urethra. She thinks, from her medical knowledge, that her symptoms have appeared following the surgery.

She makes her friend responsible for her painful intercourse and does not understand what is happening to her body, which she sees as a disgusting object, which brings us back to the first anal attachment and an image of the body as devalued and very infantile. Ariane sees the sexual act as violent and brutal, which she experienced in her relationship with her friend, especially since having cystitis. One can understand here the reaction of the body as a defence against the sex act which is not invested with libido. There is no pleasure in this act since the body sees it as an aggression and not as a pleasure. When she no does not have sex, she no longer has pain in the vulva. Then, during a session, Ariane began to remember her early childhood and talked about the ban on masturbation that her mother imposed on her when she was five years old. Her mother had been angry and had scolded her furiously. Ariane is slowly becoming aware, as part of her therapy, that her mother controls her body, even today, and that she has a way to go to become autonomous and to finally have access to pleasure. Psychically speaking, Ariane is still a child and is unable to have genital sex accompanied by pleasure.

When the patient has no bodily autonomy, it is no longer an indication of the need for psychosomatic therapies, but, rather, of psycho-corporal therapies. In the context of such therapy, after eight or ten to twelve months, patients find the way to their body, which they invest in, gradually, on the psychic plane; this then allows them to create a capacity for imagination and expressiveness: they can finally have access to a guilt-free pleasure.

After psycho-corporal therapy has restored psychosomatic unity, it is possible to continue or undertake psychosomatic therapy. The main objective is the recovery of the psychosomatic unit, the psychic investment of the organs by the libido, and, finally, access to pleasure.

CHAPTER 2

"A good enough mother"

The maternal role of the psychosomatist is strongly recommended when the patient is fixed in an archaic position of psychosexual and neuronal development. We address ourselves to the little boy or the little girl in our patients to resume the process of psychosexual maturation in relation to the neuronal process. We are in a position similar to that of our psychiatrist colleagues who work with children, although it is not identical because we are working with adults who already have extensive histories. The technique adopted is very complex, and we will describe it by first presenting a case of alcohol addiction (Elvire), then the case of a patient with a glioma (Emma).

Elvire: addiction to alcohol

In Elvire's case, I must admit that it took me a few months to understand the nature of her addiction and the role this played in the patient's psychosomatic economy.

Elvire was referred to me by a business coach just over six years ago; the exploration of Elvire's personality was long, to which must be added the establishment of a diagnosis and the elaboration of a therapeutic strategy. The nature of the fixation-regression points was not at all obvious, and it was in a relationship of apparent transference that I came to understand the psychodynamic and psychic economy of Elvire. We have come a long way in the last six years; it is this path that I will now present.

How to cure Elvire's alcohol addiction?

During these years, we have exchanged many letters, to which I will refer to gradually build the framework of the personal narrative and the psychosomatic therapy.

An initial letter that I write to her in answer to her questions:

> The road is difficult, but you have started on the way. I encourage you to continue. Work is an important part of life, and you do well, but the emotional dimension is the other essential component and we have started that work together. No one can walk this path at the speed of lightning. We must be patient. I know you suffer. You will get through this ordeal. I am at your side, and we will walk together.

Elvire describes herself as a manager working in the cultural milieu; she has important skills, and she is fully involved in her professional activities. She seems to be dominated by the way she behaves, but as we shall see later, the apparent richness of her dream life reveals an ability to think about her thoughts; although this includes significant operating deficiencies due to archaic fixations to a maternal image that has not been internalised. The problem is to define in depth the nature of the maternal image. Elvire replied very kindly to my letter:

> Your answer moves me. I agree to walk together. I know the road will be difficult, but I'll try to hold on. It's the prospect of better days that makes me want to take on this job on myself, the vision of a glimmer of hope. Thank you already for your support.

Elvire is a very intelligent patient, and she understood when I spoke about access to the unconscious and dream life. She knows it is very important if both of us are to progress. She tells me that she woke up very early in the week (at around 3am) to smoke a cigarette. She had to go back to bed because she owed me a dream. She thinks she wakes up in the night early to defend herself against dreaming, which is not at all wrong. As soon as she went back to bed, she felt great inner anguish, as if afraid of her dreams. She speaks about me as if I am some sort of external authority commanding her to dream. A relationship of the superego type seems to be being established, and it will be my task to analyse it. Elvire understands, however, that the path of dreams can lead her to progress, and she will make efforts to dream.

She dreams with images which, I will understand later, are *only* images, without any psychic working through. She shows me sensori-motor images created by daily excitations. The unconscious still seems closed off in its ability to transmit and elaborate these images at the preconscious level.

These images are a combination of her past life and the core of psychic life that is beginning to appear. She gives the first pictures the title: "baby story". She is in front of a congregation in a church, and there are at least 200 people present. She sees them as a concert hall audience, which refers to an activity she began in pre-adolescence and adolescence, when she joined an orchestra made up of teenagers. She ended up after a few years presiding over this great orchestra and I think it was an extraordinary achievement on her part.

She is standing in front of everyone, and she shows them a baby; the baby looks everyone in the eye. In the distance, he recognises a person he calls "mom". This is Elvire's mother; she goes to her mother to show her the baby.

In this sequence, Elvire appears as a baby in the first relationship to the mother. For the moment, we do not know who this mother is and what her relationship with Elvire was when she was a baby.

The dream continues twenty years later: there are four characters in this dream, namely Elvire, her sister who is the youngest of the siblings, and her older brother, and a woman appears without a face, who she identifies as the person who referred her to me, or maybe as me, the psychoanalyst.

I think here we can talk about the beginning of a pseudo-transferential relationship, but in a maternal mode: it is about a relationship of attachment, as in the first moments of life. I have significant doubts about the development of a transfer neurosis.

In pursuit of dreamlike stories, Elvire is very angry because her mother left with her brother's baby pretending that he does not know how to take care of the baby. She finds it scandalous because it is not up to her mother to decide on the baby's education. Her older brother does not react; as for her sister she seems to take the mother's side. She finds all this unacceptable, and suddenly the fourth character slaps the sister, to the satisfaction of Elvire! She feels understood.

We gradually see the appearance of the characters around Elvire, as well as the conflict situations in which she seems very isolated. The end of the dream shows that she feels understood by her therapist.

The third part of her dream shows her in the midst of people with whom she lived during her adolescence, namely young artists; they are on a huge lawn and take each other by the hand to form a huge circle. She ends up joining her colleagues and settles down as far away as she can from them, by the road, bordering the lawn, on which she lays down her head. She is therefore in danger and escapes only by getting up at the last moment so that she is not crushed by cars.

Elvire talks to me about danger, but I do not understand immediately because I still do not know about her profound addiction to alcohol. Leaving the last session, she went to have a beer, and she bought a nice necklace on the recommendation of her coach.

The problem of feminine psychic identity begins to appear in all its ambiguity. How to be a woman? What is femininity? She lived the first years of her life as a tomboy, and she carried on living in a way that privileged her masculine aspects. She returned home very late, though it usually takes less than an hour to get there. She got back very tired, and started looking in her archives, which she maintains with much care. Fifteen years ago, she was hospitalised and still retains a very bad memory of the experience. At that time, she met with a psychoanalyst who spoke with her and encouraged her; I now understand that there was some psychic work done prior to us meeting.

The psychoanalyst told her, "There was a referral error concerning you, you should never have been hospitalised." "So he thought like you," Elvire adds. "The work was not finished at the time, we will finish it together, no?" What was the reason for her hospitalisation? What exactly happened at the age of twenty? Gradually, the story of pre-adolescence and adolescence comes out as Elvire's speaks. She used to play a musical instrument and the encounter with the orchestra was very beneficial because this new universe provided her with space where she could flourish and develop. But this also had a negative aspect since at weekends the members of the orchestra gathered to binge drink together. This habit of drinking alcohol to forget everything about everyday life creates a space inside where nothing exists: no more excitations, no more tension, no more thought. Nothing.

I approached this new universe and this particular way of functioning in the context of addiction only gradually, because instead of psychic work, it is a question of all excitations turning into a sort of spasmophilia, where, through extreme anxiety, the muscles contract involuntarily. At the age of twenty, Elvire's whole world changes: she is hospitalised. She brings me a series of dreams: she is in hospital, and the doctor who has taken care of her wants to keep her for a few more days. He wants to keep her until next week and Elvire panics because she must go back to work. The doctor agrees to discharge her on condition that she comes back to the hospital later. The doctor gives her a drug in liquid form, which she drinks with much pleasure because it makes her delirious and forget her feelings: one understands that it is alcohol. She is still in the hospital, and the doctor begins to have a face: a young man whom she finds beautiful. She is lying on a rather narrow bed, which corresponds to the reality of her hospital bed. She feels a little "shot" by the drugs; she thanks the doctor and falls asleep. She returns to the hospital because the doctor made an appointment for her; and there, to her surprise, in the waiting room, is her mother! She does not know what to do; she flees without saying a word to her mother and makes an appointment with the doctor, who will call her later.

The dream reveals her relationship difficulties with her mother, then with her father; she is in "their house" and they are getting ready to eat. This is a dream about past impressions. The table is dusty, and it is obvious that the house has not been inhabited for a long time: she dusts the table, feeling deep anguish. This anguish from the past is reinforced by the appearance of his father, who is angry, he clears the whole table by showing his daughter the dust. This is the dust of the past, of her past twenty years, and of conflicts, again with her parents.

This return to the past brings back the trauma of multiple hospitalisations between the ages of twenty-two and twenty-five:

> I think, first, about this doctor at the hospital, in the emergency department. I often went there for my spasms … It's about this doctor, probably a little "perverse", a big man. Once, he locked the room I was in … I was "shot" by too much alcohol … Clinging on the bed by camisoles, stripped from head to foot by the ambulance crew … The next day, paramedics came for me, "by force", to take me to the psychiatric hospital … a traumatic journey for me … I'll have to talk about it again and again! I was treated "like an animal", deprived of my freedom … I understand that some, in such situations, go crazy … and in their madness turn their aggression against their carers … I want to do that to this doctor, because that same day, in the morning, he had taken my hand, in a caring way, at least I thought … He told me nothing about his intention to send me to the hospital shrink. I would like to discuss all of this with you again … because I think that these events strongly contribute to the resistance that I put in place in our work together. In spite of myself, in an irrational and unreasonable way, I have to fear, that in the end you do me harm …

Harm and the fear that I would hurt her gradually appear in Elvire's projections during the session. During a session, she sees, on either side of my head, two bad dogs. "I'm thinking of the two bad dogs I saw in my dreams, before our last session, those who were placed just above you, behind your armchair …" All primary associations lead to the relationship with a mother perceived as bad. Gradually, the image of the "bad mother", who accompanied all his childhood and all her adolescence, appears.

Elvire is fixed in a pre-object position to the bad mother (Melanie Klein's paranoid–schizoid position[7]) that she unconsciously seeks in all her relationships. For the moment, she can only have relations with an aggressor. There is, however, the unconscious and often very conscious, search for "this obsessional thought":

---

[7] As I explained earlier, in the paranoid–schizoid position (at the age of three months), the child gradually builds a mental representation of the primary object by cleaving the good and the bad mother. These two representations will merge around the age of nine months.

> The desire that someone take my hand, as in the song by Yves
> Duteil, which I listened to again recently, crying and sobbing
> loudly. The one I listened to tirelessly when I was a kid …
> I listening to it again this morning, I need to transcribe the
> words, for you, for me, to remember … my throat is tight, the
> tears are ready to flow again.

In this song, the words offer hope of therapeutic progress:

> Take a child by the hand,
> To take him towards tomorrow,
> To give him confidence in his footsteps.

This search for a kind maternal image, the good mother, makes me optimistic for the progress of the therapy. Above all, this points me in the direction of the cure, namely to develop the relationship with a good mother who will eventually merge with the bad mother to constitute the complete maternal object that will eventually be internalised.

Once she had recited the words of the song, Elvire added: "This is my little-girl side, and I entrust you with it now … I think you will take good care of it." She is now aware of this dimension of her personality that must be cared for in the therapeutic setting. For a therapist, this presents a heavy responsibility.

Pink Floyd and *The Wall*

We are going to slip little by little into addiction and its terrifying fantasies. One day, during a session, Elvire gave me a copy of the film *The Wall*. It is a film she used to watch over and over again, and which now, twenty years later, during the therapeutic process, she has returned to. She says, "After fifty minutes, I get fed up watching this movie … Finally, it's not me, it's *no longer* me. It's reassuring, I've changed. I'm giving you this movie, and in the end I won't miss it …"

The film is surprising because for fifty minutes there are no lyrics. Through the principal character, Pink, the film tells the story of someone locked in a hotel room somewhere in Los Angeles. He watches television in fascination at the images that appear from and disappear within the screen. We understand that this is someone who is completely wrecked by the state of his life and especially by the drugs he takes in massive amounts. Gradually, images of a violent past at the time of the Second World War appear, along with a man, a soldier, who could be his father, without this being specified. The images switch alternately from the world of war to the world of school, which is also a world where we see the violence of teacher towards students.

Reality and nightmares follow each other on the screen. Each image, each memory in the form of sensory or motor images, constitutes a "brick" in the wall that the character has gradually built around him. He is locked within a circular wall. He has built this wall to imprison his emotions. Pink slowly slides out of the world and shuts himself in a nightmare where the characters of the past attack him in an endless court case. He does not know what world he is in, and in crisis, he destroys all the objects in his hotel room. In some sense, he is destroying his inner world, which is attacking him with images that he cannot bring himself to think about. All these actions lead to the destruction of the awareness of the conscious being. This is too much sensory excitement!

The wall ends up being destroyed! Pink's fate seems to end in destruction, his gaze reflecting deep suffering and death. Pink is acting out my patient's self-destruction!

The development of the image of the "bad mother" leads to the internalisation of the cruel and violent aspect of Elvire's unconscious which, throughout her life, and until she began psychosomatic therapy, seeks out the figure of the aggressor to maintain an effective relationship of pleasure–displeasure. In Elvire's pre-adolescence and adolescence, her unconscious grasped at alcohol as if it were a door that opened into a place where consciousness vanished. Alcohol has become the internal aggressor in a world closed in on itself. Aggressive impulses turn themselves into impulses of self-destruction.

As she said, Elvire has returned, twenty years on, to this film that has for so long been part of her. In many sessions, she came back to her grandfather. In the film, we see the death of Pink's father; for her, the father she had adopted was her grandfather whom she lost when she was six years old. Her biological father was still absent; she blames him for his great dependence on his own mother, her paternal grandmother. She ended up by creating an imaginary story of her own birth.

She grew up with an "absent" father and a dead father. She has also grown up with a sick, tyrannical mother—although Elvire knows there is a lot worse. In truth, a mother who is deeply unhappy with her life.

In the film, Pink evokes harsh teachers and submissive and disciplined students, who walk in step with the music of Pink Floyd, and who end up disappearing into the void, one after the other!

For Elvire, the teachers in the film are the same as those she had from infant through to secondary school; for her, they are monsters. The deadly look of the mother at the table was the look of her mother who was terrorising her.

It is clear that the phantasmatic aspect of my patient's awareness is very important and that it will take a long time to build up the ability to see her parents, others and life in general differently. We are in a sensory world that has not yet been "thought" by the maternal relationship: still in what Bion calls the "unthought".

The students and school children in the film demonstrate how impossible it is to refuse to be put into a mould, to not conform, to not accept tyranny. Elvire tells me that she reacts against any form of tyranny and that she would even put herself in danger to do that. "I am a woman in revolt, but I am constantly restricted by this internal violence: unable to speak, I have to take the right direction … and when I let go, every time it's a catastrophe … I get it totally wrong. I get rejected."

She gradually became aware that this internal violence attracted aggression and rejection by others. This had been going on all her life, for twenty-five years.

> The condition of this suffering man's apartment is mine … not as bad, but sometimes not far off; this man who sleeps alone, it's me. This "stranger" in the world that surrounds him, with hands stretched out, this can be me when I am not well. Wanting to see no one, unable to love.
>
> On the other hand, I never remember lying down in my mother's bed … it was she who came to sleep by my side when she was not feeling well. Asking for help: "Mum is not doing

well." I could not do anything for her, I did not understand, I did not want to hold her in my arms, it scared me … her sadness. How can a little girl look after an adult woman? It is too hard.

Here are some of the lyrics of the Pink Floyd song, *Another Brick in the Wall*:

> We don't need no education
> We don't need no thought control
> No dark sarcasm in the classroom
> Teacher, leave them kids alone
> Hey, teacher, leave them kids alone
> All in all it's just another brick in the wall
> All in all you're just another brick in the wall

She returns to the film and declares:

> This man who drinks too much is me when I have too much inner pain … to lull the monster inside me; the loneliness of this man is me. After two years of therapy, I'm bored watching this movie … finally, it's not me, it's not me anymore. It's reassuring I've changed and I can give you this movie without regret, finally, I will not miss it. The only positive thing is that the wall falls at the end. At the time I did not understand these images, the "message" … the wall the man had locked himself inside of, collapses, brick after brick. This is me … I feel relieved.

It must be understood that this was a long journey of controlling the alcohol; it took almost two years for her to wean herself off it. Withdrawal, for an addict, is an extended ordeal; we trod this challenging path together. I was not a victim of my narcissism (countertransference) because I quickly realised that I could not achieve this weaning alone. I thought it important to also use a group, in this case, Alcoholics Anonymous, which could support the patient and help her engage in the process. Elvire kindly followed my advice and contacted this organisation.

She knew very well that alcohol was destroying her from the inside. She was suffering from it but could not shake off its grip.

She made several resolutions, which she wrote down and sent to me:

> I pledge to stop drinking as of … My reasons for stopping are: this poison rots my life, I do not love myself so it prevents me from functioning normally, I jeopardise my professional future even though I have great abilities; I exhaust myself stupidly, I waste a lot of time and money, money I need. I want to live and stop destroying myself; I cut myself off from the world, from all social life … which just makes my loneliness worse. To get ready to stop drinking, here are the things I'm going to do: play sports, read, read, and read again, find pleasure by any other means that do not endanger my health.

As she had feared, coming off the alcohol took us a good two years, accompanied by episodes that were often dramatic. Elvire told me about here about the five anti-relapse rules:

> Stay motivated, make a list of the benefits of having stopped drinking alcohol; avoid taking even a glass; prepare an emergency plan in case alcohol is consumed again, especially avoid drinking again regularly, do not buy alcohol, and in the event of relapse, analyse the reasons for drinking; do not criticise myself too much, call on the help of your relatives; if you experience withdrawal symptoms, consult my regular doctor or therapist; always analyse relapses to avoid risk situations.

Appearance of masochism

Addiction to alcohol has gradually replaced the "bad maternal image", and in the transference relationship this has gradually become established: Elvire sees me as the ally of her mother and criticises me for it. She found herself an abuser, a substitute for her mother. But that does not last, because we have to make progress. She will gradually become aware that she has internalised the aggressor and that the phenomenon of self-destruction is at work. While well understanding the direction of the cure, she suffers from extreme privation. She can no longer attack the awareness from which she wants to escape.

> I am still writing to you because I am not well, I will kill them all. I do not like my parents, I do not like my brother, I do not like my sister; they all made me suffer and they do not even realise it! I do not feel well in this family, they spend their time making me feel guilty for not being theirs.

Elvire is not yet in an ambivalent relationship and continues to cling to the images of "good" and "bad".

Her lucidity begins to appear:

> Hello Professor Stora, yes, you're right, I slipped further, deeply. I think I actually understood what you told me but I guess it suits me to let you believe the opposite through my letters, distort your words and play the injured one. It's really mean as behaviour; we will talk about it quietly tomorrow even if I am a little ashamed. Today, I woke up with the desire to cry about all my nonsense, but I told myself that my childishness had lasted long enough and that I now have to invest in life and stop locking myself in the pleasure of displeasure. I still have to live without you, it will be very difficult, but you helped me yesterday. I dreamed, I will tell you, that I think we are not at the end of our troubles. As you say, my problem is really "archaic", my problem is to accept and integrate the idea of having the right to live, for myself, for my pleasure and without causing displeasure to others … in any case, without making myself feel guilty.

Elvire has made a lot of progress, and the love of maternal attachment (love of the young child for her mother) appears in all her letters, which is a very positive sign of the progressive development of the infantile neurosis. We have already come a very long way.

All this is confirmed in a letter in which Elvire first recalls her values, which she attributes to me: friendship, complicity, exchange, listening, understanding, comfort, mutual help, joy, and happiness. "It has been," she says:

> my model for life for twenty-five years now. I find this model in you; I still need a teacher in my life, and I know, more than ever,

that I found it in you! For you are a kind man, who sympathises with my misfortunes; you are not dogmatic and you do not seek to impose your laws upon me; you respect my personality and you help me to express it … I wish you well. Our work … gives me a lot of hope that I will live …

Elvire has brilliantly illustrated the work of the psychosomatist therapist and the psychoanalyst.

Return of the libido

In psychosomatics we know that somatic energy and libidinal energy are strongly activated by disease. The return of the libido is a very positive sign of the arousal of the life drive and therefore an improvement in the health of patients. Gradually, in a series of dreams, the oedipal conflict and romantic relationships appear:

I knock on the door of my father's room and ask him if I can return to use the room next door to change. I see my father in a nice, young man's suit, with a trendy tie. He repeats a scene where he posed as a playboy for the evening. And he said to me, "I told them I will not drink, but I think I'll let myself be tempted." I wanted to tell him not to do it because if he starts, he will not be able to stop. And he will be completely wasted. I change my mind, […]; and finally, I say to myself: […] after all, he is not me. The others will not judge me through him; there is no reason for me to reject him. In any case, I'm sure, I will not let myself be tempted. And I tell my dad that I'm going to change in the next room.

The following dreams are more explicit about the oedipal conflict. Since the beginning of the therapy, Elvire had had no identification with women; she lived as a boy, and later a young man who hated women. Having spent many years alone with her brother in front of the television, Elvire took Superman as an ideal.

The series of dreams reported shows very clearly the evolution and psychic object structuring of progress towards genitality. The main problem appears, then, to have a feminine psychic identification.

The neurological dimension of addiction

If we only think of addiction in psychic terms, we have not done all our work, because the pleasure centres of the central nervous system will continue to act by trying to unbalance the psychic system. The central nervous system has very complex centres of reward and pleasure, and our work must gradually move onto the level of the pleasure centres.

The role of the brain's reward circuit allows the brain to assign a positive craving to a consumed substance or behaviour. We talk about positive reinforcement that facilitates the repetition of the behaviour.

> This reward circuit is a very phylogenetically conserved system and one of the assumptions is that drugs only usurp a natural system involved in positive reinforcement. The problem is that the drugs activate this system in a powerful way, in comparison with the natural reinforcing agents, by modifying the efficiency of the interneuronal transmission: "the synaptic plasticity", which appears as the neurobiological substrate explaining the mechanisms of learning and memorisation.
>
> (Naassila & Pierrefiche, 2018)

We talk about the "pathological memory" of addiction, with long-term traces in the brain explaining the possibility of relapse long after consumption has ceased. Professor Naassila explains:

> At the beginning of the addiction, the positive reinforcement predominates. The reward system adjusts in such a way that the threshold of reward-effects increases. But the sensation deficit of the positive effects makes an effort to take advantage of the substance. Then chronic exposure leads to disturbances in certain brain structures so that the positive reinforcement will give way to a negative reinforcement.
>
> (Naassila & Pierrefiche, 2018)

In other words, the processes of neuro-adaptation adjust themselves in order to make a disruption, and drugs that are powerful enough lead to the establishment of opposing "anti-reward" processes that aim to accurately counter a superactivation of this reward system. Other neurotransmitters will come into play and explain the implementation of negative reinforcement. The subject will no longer consume the substance just to feel its positive effects, but also to relieve the negative effects—that is to say, the unpleasant sensations that occur during weaning, physical or mental, and urge for the substance to be consumed again. This balance between positive and negative craving (this insatiable desire) leads to the maintenance of the level of consumption of the substance despite its negative effects: loss of control and compulsive taking of the product. We begin to understand the dysfunctions of the brain in addictions, especially at the level of the reward circuit, represented by the nucleus accumbens (ventral striatum, a substructure of the striatum) which receives afferences from the ventral tegumentary area. The nucleus accumbens is invaded by dopamine during the consumption of substances, which gives rise to a feeling of pleasure: the dopamine serves, in part, to attribute an added value that is perceived during the consumption of a substance or as a result of behaviour. It is also used to encode more complex phenomena, such as prediction errors when receipt of a drug is expected but does not take place.

Thus, the product intake is directed initially towards the search for positive effects, and then the behaviour ends up switching to an automatic mode. In addition, the nucleus accumbens is under the control of other brain structures, such as the hippocampus, which sends excitatory glutamatergic afferents. However, the hippocampus is involved in the process of memorisation, and memory plays an important role in this reward circuit (memorisation of the intensity of the sensations, the context in which the product is consumed) and therefore a major role in the phenomenon of relapse. In other words, the commitment of a subject to a compulsive, repetitive, automatic behaviour is linked to the fact that the brain structures involved in negative reinforcement play a preponderant role, and also with the lifting of the inhibition normally exerted in the cortical regions. We now understand better that it is not just drugs that precipitate relapse and govern consumption; environmental factors, negative emotional states, and dysphoria also play an important role in negative reinforcement. This is why, Professor Naassila insists, a drug addict is in such a state of discomfort that, unconsciously, his only way to relieve himself is to take the product. This subject has lost control; when he is addicted, he does not even know why he consumes the substance.

It is important to review the various steps that Elvire must take before approaching the neuronal weaning stage. In the first stage, we were in the presence of pathological manifestations caused by her addiction: drinking until losing consciousness, reaching the "nothing"; in the sessions, projections in a hallucinatory mode where terrifying parental images appeared. This makes one fear for the weaknesses of the ego if the psychotic core were to come to the surface. All the material of the sessions referred to the archaic sensorimotor fixations explaining the use of addictive dependence: alcohol and cigarettes, and thus the absence of the mother. The anamnesis with past–present round trips revealed a satisfactory functioning potentiality of the psychic system; dreams that she had enable us to discover a very rich imagination. The preconscious seemed solid and well-constituted.

The second stage was spread over the years 2012 and 2013 during which internalisation of the object progressively took place: the psychosomatist as a temporary maternal image. We were able to access this stage after having interpreted the masochistic dimension in the relationship with the aggressor; a terrifying maternal image of the first years of life was replaced in adolescence by self-destructive, addictive dependency.

This was followed by a stage of ambivalent reconciliation with her mother and her father, of the restoration of emotional bonds which allowed the patient to see the birth of her desire for withdrawal (the coexistence of maternal images: Elvire's mother and the therapist), and, eventually, the internalisation of the maternal image of Elvire's mother. I was only able to take up the delicate weaning procedure after I had Elvire agree to attend a group at the same time to fight the addiction to alcohol. I would like to remind you that for the therapist to undertake such a process of withdrawal on his own is a very risky enterprise. The first four months were extremely difficult; there were many incidents, including hospitalisations.

Thanks to therapeutic support, the deep desire of the patient, and the help of members of the alcohol control group, Elvire was able to engage in weaning and resist her desire to drink. For my part, I provided continuous encouragement.

Therapeutic and neurological work

The therapeutic and neurological work was done at the level of the pleasure principle, to find sources of satisfaction to compensate for, and replace, in time, the pleasure of drinking to the point of losing consciousness: that is, a reorientation of Eros and the life instincts. This psychic work was accompanied, progressively over a period of approximately nine to eighteen months, by neuronal modifications intended to re-establish a satisfactory neurological functioning to allow a return to "positive reinforcement".

We continue psychosomatic psychotherapy with the appearance of the unresolved oedipal conflict in adolescence. Elvire copes with the gaps between sessions and her frustration. She can mentalize absence and resist frustration; she does not write to me between sessions. Weaning can only be considered definitive once the neurological consolidation has happened, and this, in my clinical experience, will take between nine and eighteen months. In truth, there can be perfectly successful weaning only if the functioning of the neurological structures, unbalanced by the addiction, has been re-established. Psychotherapy has facilitated the emergence of a superego nucleus and the resurgence of an orbitofrontal control on which the patient relies to resist the insatiable desire to drink. She does not want to trouble me or hurt her father, her mother, her brother, her sister. A psychic and neuronal control appears.

Psychosomatic therapy continues in psychoanalytic psychotherapy since we are going to tackle the oedipal conflict and we are going to shift into a world that is very different from that of the previous years.

Theoretical clarifications

I prefer to present the details of the theoretical underpinning of the approach here, at the end of the presentation of this case. As Bion has very clearly explained to us, there is originally an unthinking thought, a thought that does not have the ability to think. At first, there are only sensations and motor behaviours, things in themselves, what Sigmund Freud calls representations of things and that Bion calls beta-elements in a word, the unthinkable.

The role of the mother is that of what Bion calls the alpha-function, which transforms beta-elements into thought. It is with the alpha-function that we put words onto things. Our role as a psychosomatist in the imaginary void of our patients is to fulfil this alpha-role and to gradually develop a device with which to think thoughts. In this way, the external and internal excitations are progressively taken over by this apparatus which is, along with the immune system, an important system of defence of the psychosomatic unit.

Let us now turn to Winnicott who has been for me in the last twenty-five years a master and a guide in my therapeutic approach. In "Fear of breakdown" (1974), he declares:

> The individual proceeds from absolute dependence to relative independence and towards independence. In health, the development takes place at a pace that does not outstrip the development of complexity in the mental mechanisms, this being linked to neuro-physiological development … The facilitating environment can be described as *holding*, developing into *handling*, to which is added *object-presenting* … In such a facilitating environment the individual undergoes development which can be classified as *integrating*, to which is added *in-dwelling* (or *psycho-somatic collusion*) and then *object-relating* … At the time of absolute dependence, with the mother supplying an auxiliary ego-function, it has to be remembered that the infant has not yet separated out the "not-me" from the "me"—this cannot happen apart from the establishment of the "me."
>
> (Winnicott, 1974, p. 104, original emphasis)

We thus have the therapeutic approach necessary to help our somatic patients who are fixed in the archaic phases of development. The main objective is to develop the device to think thoughts, to facilitate the development, reinforcement, and integration of the ego and at the same time gradually introduce the internalisation of the maternal object.

All of this, as Winnicott says, is very difficult, time-consuming, and painful, but at least it is not futile.

Emma: a brain-damaged patient injured and the maternal role in the neurological field

I present here the psychosomatic approach of a patient operated on for a glioma: this is the neurological disorder Emma lives with.

In psychosomatics, we have developed two approaches to disease: the illness as seen by the doctor and the illness as experienced by the patient. We also ask ourselves what role is performed by the disease in the psychosomatic balance of the patient?

What is Emma suffering from after her brain surgery on a glioma which took place a year ago? Following her operation, Emma suffered from aphasia and epileptic seizures every two or three weeks, often in the evening; she has long periods of insomnia. Emma has a foreign accent, a mixture of English and German intonation. She tells me that after the operation she spoke for a while in English and could no longer speak French. The limits of remembering words and actual experiences have been reached. She experiences emotions that I feel strongly and immediately during the sessions. I then communicate to her what I feel, which she confirms: an emotion of distress, especially due to her condition and her inability to readily make use of her previous rich vocabulary.

Sometimes she seemed very robotic and sometimes very human in her desire to recover her verbal ability. She reads books; she remembers the atmosphere and environment of the book, but not the characters or what they say to each other. She was very tired in the first sessions; her daytime fatigue is often caused by epileptic seizures that occur at night. She has not dreamed since last year; before her operation, she had a lot of anxiety dreams. Her memory, since the operation, is more auditory than visual. She remembers everything she hears, but not what she reads in books: she takes notes but cannot remember which part of the book they are taken from; nor can she watch a film, because she does not understand all the words she hears and cannot follow the action of the characters. She offered me a book on neuropsychology, in which she had annotated many passages, including the following. About his patient, Zazetsky, "the man with a shattered world", Alexander Luria (1972) writes:

> He could no longer understood the logic, cause and effect, or
> spatial relationships. He couldn't distinguish his left from his
> right … He couldn't comprehend a whole word, understand
> a sentence or recall a complete memory because doing any of
> these things would require relating symbols. He could grasp
> only fleeting fragments.

Emma's operation had caused a disturbance of her ability to hear words, to assemble them, to make them into intelligible sentences, and to retain everything.

Emma also tells me about the loss of language automatisms: when she speaks with people at the library, she cannot remember all the questions they ask her; she only retains the first question and attempts a response. In addition, language automatisms such as hello, goodbye, Happy New Year, etc. seem to fail her. She cannot use them quickly; she must think about it first. She knows the meaning of the words but cannot use them in conversation. She used to love punk music, but now the music is a noise she is incapable of interpreting.

Emma's story

Emma is a slender young woman with brown hair, who stares at me with a look that, at first, I think is questioning, but during the session will suddenly, and frequently, reveal itself to be quite vacant. When she was young she was a great reader—of fairy tales, but especially the books that were in her school classroom; her mother also brought her books to read from the library. Emma now works in the local library.

She tells me that her mother is aggressive towards her and her sisters, that her condition is psychiatric. I tell her that it may be a character trait that has been interpreted as a psychiatric disorder, but, without explaining the circumstances, she tells me that her mother has, at some point, been detained in hospital.

At the age of seventeen, Emma left her family to go to Paris, first to study literature, then to be a librarian. She is now thirty-eight years old and lives with a young man called Maurice who was her work colleague.

It all started in September 2007, when she collapsed after what could have been an epileptic seizure, and then coma ensued. She returned to work in December 2007, and in March 2008 she was operated on for a glioma. She went back to work again at the end of June. Her sister Clarice currently lives with her daughter in the South of France. As for Emma's father, whom she calls a "sympathetic stranger", he has apologised to her for having been silent all these years. During the session, she equates the attitude of her father to that of the French who, during the war, just watched as trains were filled with Jews being deported. She has integrated the climate of violence in which she lived and grew up throughout her childhood. Her mother beat the three little girls violently. Although we cannot blame this conflictual behaviour for the glioma, we can pay attention to the masochistic dimension of the situation.

We can then understand Emma's escape into drugs. From the age of twelve, with one of her girlfriends, she started smoking marijuana and drinking alcohol, and this lasted until she met Maurice. She stopped drinking alcohol at the age of twenty-four; as for marijuana, she continues to smoke from time to time. She still smokes a lot of cigarettes. She thinks that her sister, Clarice, and she were gifted children because they had outstanding grades at school up until the *baccalaureate*, although there were many subjects that did not interest her. She cycles every day; previously it had been very long distances, hundreds of kilometres. She also practices an Asian combat sport at a club near her home. Because of her brain surgery and the fear of traumatic shock possibly causing an epileptic fit, she has given up combat sports. Since the age of fourteen she has been vegetarian and has maintained such a diet for more than twenty years. Her mother, and her two sisters, cooked for her. Her mother was not a great cook, but she took care of her children, and despite Emma's criticism of her, the image of an ambivalent mother, absorbed by her high school teaching profession and the education of her three daughters, gradually emerged.

Emma lived until the age of ten in the South of France and after went to the north of the country where her mother was a teacher in a high school; it was very difficult for her because her accent was made fun of, and it took her two years to adapt. She was the first in the class, but this changed when she attended the most important high school in her city, an elitist school which selected students by exam. The adaptation was difficult for her. Until her surgery, she was happy with her work at the library.

The therapeutic process: twenty-five therapy sessions over eight months

At the beginning the interviews were chaotic because, if I did not ask questions and did not lead the conversation, Emma would just stare at me in silence. Whenever I did not speak the silence returned, and when I asked her "What are you thinking about?" She replied, "Nothing." Unlike the many classical patients of psychoanalysis who are in a state of repression and fixed in an oedipal genital position, Emma really did think of nothing; it was an absence of thought, as with many somatic patients whose pathologies are archaic and pregenital.

I then adopted the psychosomatic method developed at the Pitié-Salpêtrière Hospital with my patients, that is to say:

1. Gradually build into the therapeutic relationship the links between words, emotions, and thoughts, current thoughts, and thoughts of the patient's past: in this particular case, work on the recovery of semantic memory and mental and emotional representations of her past.
2. In psychosomatic therapy, we play the role of a benevolent and empathetic mother reactivating the baby's first invested relationship with the mother; it is not, as in the classical cure of psychoanalysis, a question of transference. Such a maternal attitude facilitates identification with the psychotherapist who becomes a caring and empathetic maternal image: a mirror of the patient or parent. It is an attachment relationship.

During the sessions, Emma experienced emotions that I felt strongly and instantly: emotions mostly related to her condition and her inability to quickly mobilise the rich vocabulary which she had been accustomed to use in her past. Therapeutically, since Emma was unable to mobilise her thoughts to talk to me, I began to ask her about her vocation, her curiosity about books, her studies, and her current work: the technique I developed in psychosomatics to facilitate the establishment of connections between mental representations, emotions, and behaviours. This technique activates and contributes to the construction of associative chains.

She tries to recover very slowly her previous mental and verbal abilities. According to my experience in the organ transplantation department, it takes nine to eighteen months for new synaptic connections to develop. It seems that the neuropsychologist and the speech therapist told Emma it would take about two years. In the sessions, through the use of metaphor, I attempt to stimulate her imaginative and auditory abilities.

She has been dreaming for several sessions and I choose the following dream: she is in her bed, in her room; a woman is standing there and lifting up the duvet, showing Emma a cardboard box in which are stored the tiny bodies of five children of different sizes. In the session preceding this dream, Emma had brought me a lot of drawings she had done over the last fifteen years; I had encouraged her to resume this activity so that the right hand, which had been impaired by the brain surgery, could practice some activity. I also advised her, in the same session, to talk openly with her colleagues about the disruption to her work that the surgery was creating.

Interpretation of the dream

I began by drawing her attention to the five bodies, assuming that they represented her hand, the five fingers of her hand. Emma cannot associate for the moment, but gradually she began to understand the use of metaphorical language: the "five fingers of the hand" had been locked up in a cardboard box. She had ended up thinking that it was not the time to start drawing again; hence the five fingers stored in an unusable cardboard box. She accepted my interpretation, telling me that for the moment she was tired and could not pick it up again.

Emma sits timidly on the edge of the armchair and looks at me questioningly because she expects everything from me; she looks at me like a child looking at the mother who will take the initiative to talk to her, to teach her things in life. For her, I must be the mirror of her thoughts and the feelings of her thoughts, so that she can rebuild herself.

We then go on to investigate what technical device could help her to remember because the information comes to her through visual and auditory sensory pathways that seem to be affected, which prevents the process of neural encoding for remembering. Emma confirms this hypothesis and I think then the only way to remember is to go through the motor pathways: she is to take notes on small sheets for each book she is reading and, this way, she will remember with her fingers what she has read. She confirms that when she writes, she remembers what she has read. Together, we decide that she will use this technique: she will write the summaries on small sheets that she will put in a box. Thus, she will be able to answer the library users' questions who ask for information on new books.

In the therapeutic interview, I only use short sentences expressing only one thought at a time. I also decide to conduct the sessions with questions addressing all aspects of her current life in order to accustom her to evoking more and more current memories and to create in her working memory the associative capacities, first, between events in a particular context (for example, her working world), then developing the ability to make links between different areas of her everyday life so that she can move faster and faster from one to the other.

For example, when I asked her about her reading, taking care not hurt her with questions that might draw attention to the fact that she does not remember what she has read, she tells me that what she has read recently makes her think about cold. I have noted several times that she attaches great importance to the atmosphere and "climate" of a book, and that she never speaks to me about the characters in the book. I associate myself then with the current cold of the winter period that we are going through, and I evoke the cold of the city of her parents in which she lived by telling her that certainly, it was much colder than in Paris. She hates the cold, and it allows her to start associating on her life.

The drawing out, by herself, of these events, of what she felt, the back and forth between the past and the present, allows me to think that the beginning of associative work, an objective that I have pursued since the beginning of this therapy, is very modestly being realised. I congratulate Emma for the accomplishment of this work and her newly acquired abilities.

Narcissistic valorisation and reconstitution of psychosomatic unity after four months of therapeutic treatment

In another session, I remember Emma's initial hostile silence towards me, as if she were disturbed by my questions, which have only one goal: to help her start the associative chains allowing her to recover good psychic functioning. She looks at me and ends up telling me that my questions are disturbing her and that she does not want to talk to me. I then understand that we are in a relationship where a hostile emotion (appearance of the negative) arises in a repetition of behaviours. I then ask her who she usually acts out with in this way and she answers me, in a kind manner, that it's about her mother and she does not want to answer her questions. I change things then by explaining the reason for my work with her and the therapeutic goals we are pursuing. I try to differentiate between the maternal relationship and the therapeutic relationship. She now better understands what I'm saying, and therefore my intention; she responds by evoking a painful point in her past which refers to the present situation, namely, not to trust the other person. She tells me about the death by suicide of an intimate friend named Janine, whom she knew when she was in second grade, and who died at the age of twenty-two. Emma revealed her feelings of guilt towards her deceased friend, because it had been at the time of Janine's death that she had met her current boyfriend, and the new investment in a relationship had taken her away from her friend. She felt guilty for having abandoned her. This is a session where there was significant abreaction.

Therapeutic progress

At the tenth session, she reminds me that she has epileptic seizures only once a week or once every two weeks and that, in most cases, the epileptic seizure happens at home. I ask her if her body sends her a warning signal before the crisis, and how she interprets such a signal. She ended up noting that shortly before the crisis, her eyesight becomes blurred and that the crisis ensues an hour later, which allows her to lie down in bed so that it can happen without any accidents. This lucidity concerning the relationship with her body is a favourable factor for the progress of the therapy as I can see that she is listening to her body.

She loves punk music, and she is now able to listen to it: until now, the music had been just a noise she could not make sense of, it was just a sound. The fact that she can give meaning to what she hears in the musical field informs me of a probable evolution of synaptic connections. It is obvious that the therapeutic sessions have succeeded in developing a sonic protective shield—the "sound envelope" of Didier Anzieu (1989, pp. 157–173)—which favoured the synaptic development of sensory cortex of hearing, sensory listening, and harmonisation of these sounds so that they do not constitute an attack on the somatic self and the psychic self.

In the twentieth session, there is the disappearance of Anglo-German intonation and the resumption of a good maternal image. Emma seems today much more alive and available in the relationship than before; she smiles, and her slight Germanic accent has practically disappeared. The flow of speech is faster, and Emma seems to quickly access words and expressions. She tells me that she had a dream, and she starts the session by talking to me about it. She is in a very large apartment that she does not know and all her family are there, reunited: her sister Suzanne, her sister Clarice, who will come soon to Paris, her mother, and her father, feet under the table (as usual, he's a perfect, solicitous, stranger). This dream is some sort of family reconciliation. Emma, happy, will make a cake and starts making the batter. But her mother tastes it and declares that it is not sweet enough. Emma is unhappy and leaves. The dream continues with her paternal grandmother whom she loves very much and who died about four years ago. In her dream, she wants to find a mother figure she can love; she does not wish to see her mother again, she tells me, and seems quite categorical about this. My maternal role must now change. Her psychic apparatus has found a maternal image.

Emma recently took pleasure in reading—something that had disappeared after her operation. She also now likes meeting her group of friends, listening to rock music. After twenty-five sessions of psychosomatic therapy, Emma has changed a lot and I would like to summarise the important points and the progress she has made.

First, the rate at which can speak has increased considerably; it seems that she is quickly accessing most common vocabulary. Second, her Anglo-Germanic accent has disappeared and synaptic connections have restored her French intonation; this point was also noted by the psycho-neurologist. Third, she is comfortable in her body, crosses the space without any difficulty, and sits in her chair smiling.

I ask her if she knows she is much better; she answers me with a smile and approves the diagnosis because, she declares, thanks to the flow of the words she has found, she has been able to restore friendly and social relations and break out of her isolation. She also tells me that she no longer takes notes to remember the books she can now recommend to readers. She thinks it's the work we're doing that has helped improve her current state. I tell her that the work we do goes in two directions, and that she has been truly involved in it.

She tells me one last dream: she is with her epileptologist, whom she knows, but his face is black; he asks her to wait a bit because, he says, from his window he can watch the parking lot where there are cars. Her dream ends there, she does not understand it.

I try to get her involved by offering associative channels: to monitor the parking in such a residence may mean that we are in a dangerous suburb; did she live in such a suburb? Yes, she tells me it was ten years ago, in her hometown. Her doctor's black face may reflect a darkening of her health at that time, and she tells me that perhaps the glioma had begun to develop during those years. She informs me in this regard that gliomata grow at a rate of 8 per cent per year.

In conclusion, I think of the very beginning of our work, of her hesitant approach, her difficulties in verbal expression, and how it is the reverse of what is happening now, like a reflection in a mirror. Today I find that I am not tired at the end of the session, as I have been in previous sessions. I invent a new concept: "the good enough mirror".

CHAPTER 3

Serious illness and pain

Béatrice: breast cancer

In psychosomatism, as in medicine, we, unlike our psychoanalyst colleagues, are confronted with serious diseases and death. In 1985, when I joined Dr Pierre Marty at the Institute of Psychosomatics, I became familiar, very quickly, with the incidence of, and the issues around, breast cancer. Pierre Marty himself was engaged in research that was later published in England. So, at that time, I started to develop therapeutic relationships with patients suffering from such a pathology.

As part of my consultation at the Pitié-Salpêtrière, I began to receive breast cancer patients because in 2008 I had started research on this pathology and a colleague gynaecologists referred patients to me. My research was completed in 2017 and the article (2018) summarising the results and commenting on patient cases appeared in the *Integrative Psychosomatic Journal*.

Meeting with Béatrice

Thus, in December 2008, I met Béatrice: I can remember very well this patient that I followed for nearly eight years in psychosomatic therapy, first in the hospital and then in private practice. Béatrice begins immediately to talk to me about her "Claude Bernard Horner syndrome", namely ptosis of the left eye; she worries a lot about it because—and this has been confirmed throughout the time I have devoted to her—she experiences any attack on her body—including in relation to her breast cancer, which has recently returned and which is causing much anxiety—as a profound narcissistic injury.

I learn, within minutes, about the recurrence of breast cancer, but I do not know what it really is: I do not know anything about her experience before breast cancer and I do not know anything about the cancer itself or why it has recently returned.

Béatrice attaches great importance to her appearance; however, there is no desire for seduction, either in an archaic mode (in relation to the mother) or in a genital mode. It is about the relationship with herself and the image she wants to give herself. From the beginning of our interview, there appears to be great fragility and distress linked to numerous events that she is currently living through with difficulty. The ptosis dates from November 2008, and the many tests done to monitor the cancer have all been negative. She continues to speak about the problem with her eye; she had blamed it on a beauty product she has used on her face, but this has turned out not to be the case. A scan she recently had tells her that everything is fine.

Here we see a hypochondriac dimension linked to the threat of breast cancer. Any sensory perception triggers the thought of a threat. She begins the story of a cancer in the left breast that dates from 1991: a tumour 5cm in diameter, followed by chemotherapy, radiotherapy, and then brachytherapy, lasting from November 1991 to June 1992. In July 1996, nodules appeared; they were operated on in 1997; then the removal of the left breast. This operation was followed, until March 1998, by chemotherapy. I gradually have a table of medical events that will accompany our therapy for many years.

In 2002 there was another discovery of nodules, this time nine of them; today there are five left. Béatrice is a member of a breast cancer patient group; she sometimes reports to me during our interviews some of the exchanges that she has in this group. She says to me, "I love life like Scarlett O'Hara in *Gone with the Wind*; I love gardening, my father taught me." She lives in a house in the suburbs where she has a kitchen garden that she cannot look after at the present time, because it is winter. This garden, which she will describe to me in other sessions, will take on considerable importance in the therapy.

She returns to a fear of being late for her appointments: "I hate arriving late," she says. In fact, that day, the commuter train was late, and she was afraid of not being on time for the session. She begins to tell me about her husband with whom she does not really get along: "He does not support me." Her husband has always been anxious about his wife's cancer, not wanting to know anything; his name is Henri. They have been married since 1970; she was twenty-three years old at the time. In a few words, Béatrice describes a difficult relationship with a husband whose obsessive traits have shown themselves little by little during the marriage. A fortnight ago her husband Henri was unwell; I personally think it was a problem with the vagal nerve, because his electrocardiogram was good. Henri is sixty-three years old; at that time, he was suffering from diarrhoea. I feel deeply all Béatrice's emotions relating to her difficulties in her life with Henri.

She is living with a husband who does not support her emotionally, totally locked in an obsessional pathology; it seems to me, however, despite Béatrice's complaints, that she has the mental capacity to keep her relationship with Henri at a distance. She suffers narcissistically, but not excessively. She changes theme, and therefore the associative chain, addressing a professional problem. Her ability to gradually address the different aspects of her life makes me suspect that Béatrice has good psychic functioning.

She had been working in a film production company and I suddenly realise that professional events were decisive in the shock that her psychic apparatus had experienced, and its somatic vulnerability. She was fired when she was fifty-one; when we met at the hospital, she was sixty-one years old. At the time of the firing, she was undergoing chemotherapy for breast cancer, and she sees it as a sign from above, because it meant she was able to think about her life and what was happening to her.

But everything had started much earlier, since in 1991 her service in the company was closed; she was the only one to be kept on. She volunteered to go to other services, and she said, "I've been through hell." One can think of all this organisational violence accompanying the dismissal procedures: "I lived six months of hell. Afterward, we had to find a post." She became responsible for managing filming operations. "I never stopped," she says, "except in the chemotherapy period." We can assume, by reconstructing the history, that not everything happened in 1991 and that there were many other sources of tension and of stress at work and, perhaps, in the family before that date. Béatrice lived in a highly stressful professional environment, and she was a victim because, gradually, when the mental apparatus is taken aback, it is the immune defences that are put under strain for a few years before decompensation and onset of serious illness.

Béatrice is now addressing the spiritual dimension of her life: she grew up in a practicing Catholic family; she prays in church. She has this resource, which, in my view, is very important in making her aware of her own resilience. She speaks to me about her two parents, and there are tears (she also cried when she spoke, at the beginning, about the investigation of her ptosis). Her mother died in August 2004 from colon cancer, she was eight-two years old; Béatrice is crying profusely, and it is obvious that mourning her mother is still going on. In this respect, the excitations connected with the loss of the maternal object are still feeding the disease. As for her father, he has just gone back into hospital; he is ninety-two, and she describes him as a lucid and courageous being.

She loves her father. She is very anxious because the surgeons have proposed a surgical operation whose outcome is uncertain. It is a risky operation for a very elderly man and, on several occasions during the session, she asks me for my opinion regarding the surgical indication, and I reply by saying that in the case of patients of very advanced age I recommend not operating. It is a responsibility that I take on, and have always taken on in the hospital, often in the face of hostility on the part of some, but not all, surgeons. In this regard, I must say, to my great surprise, that doctors are often very poor with patients aged eighty and over!

I advise Béatrice to spend time with her father so that he can be surrounded by affection for as long as is possible. She has a sister born in 1943; Béatrice was born in 1947. The two sisters have an older brother who lives far away, in the South of France. She describes him as a "marginal being". She reviews all the recent incidents: mourning her mother, her father's heart problems, her husband's problems, and she tells me that this causes her trouble: colitis and stomach upset. We understand that the excitations caused by all these dramas are not due solely to activity of the mental apparatus. The anxieties seem of very high intensity, and impossible to manage: it is a somatic alarm signal. In psychosomatics, this is called "acute irregularities of mental functioning".

She then returns to her in-laws: she loves her father-in-law who died, and her mother-in-law who died in 1998. On these two deaths, she discovered "a lot of things" about her husband. He had grown up in an apartment where, throughout his childhood and adolescence, he had no place to sleep. He therefore slept in the dining room where there was a couch that was opened every night and closed in the morning. He never had a room of his own, he grew up with a very obsessive mother, and he still today behaves in such a way in their house, where he tries to control everything.

Béatrice's vital resources

She speaks, at this point, of all the activities that occupy her while her husband stays in, has no friends, and has no plans for life. She has a "Friends of the Louvre Card", and she visits the museum regularly. She takes classes at the Sorbonne ("Where does humanity go?", history classes, courses on the history of cabinet making …) and she plays sports and belongs to a hiking club. We understand better, then, her psychic functioning because there is a very good use of psychic and vital energy. Béatrice has important resources that can ensure her survival and defence against breast cancer. She can invest her libidinal and somatic energy in many activities, which can limit the development of the cancer. Béatrice has very good mental defences.

We go back to her past and she recognises that, since 1974, the time of the restructuring of her company, she has lived with anxiety, because every two years there were redundancies. We understand the climate of professional stress in which she lived all these years, accompanied by tensions in her marriage. Professional stress throughout her career but, at the same time, exceptional psychic resistance.

I wonder about the traumas of her childhood and she reveals to me that at the age of ten, while she was with her grandparents in Vichy, she witnessed the assassination of a senator; she was walking in the street with her family, behind a group of people, when suddenly hooded men appeared and fired on the senator, wounding a woman. She lost 3 kilograms in the night. She was panicked by having witnessed this assassination; she remembers that her grandfather did not understand her emotional state, had slapped her. Since then, she has slept badly; she dreams that she is going to be killed by one of the masked men because she has witnessed the assassination. She keeps a small light, a night light, turned on every night in her room. She is afraid of violence.

She then remembers that her mother told her that at the age of nine months she had had pneumonia and almost died. She weighed 15 kilograms at the age of six. I am wondering about "early anorexic" behaviour and difficult relationships with food. Shifting from her mother to her father, she associates on an idyllic image: she went to collect chestnuts with her father and took very long walks in the forest. We end on the relationship with her father, and I propose that we meet again to explore his life a little more.

She gets up and asks me to confirm what I told her about her father because she needs reassurance; she is inhabited by very strong emotion, squeezes my hand very tightly between her hands and gives me a kiss. We end the session with intense emotion. She seems grateful for the welcome I have given her and for our interview. I suddenly remember that at another time and in another country, Sigmund Freud was confronted at the hospital by a patient threw herself into his arms, and I still laugh at his horrified reaction!

A first evaluation

The potential threat is, at present, in the home environment. She has mental development and life-event management skills that can help her withstand what is happening. Béatrice is fixed in an oedipal conflict, and all the relations of the first sessions show important capacities of mental defences. Her ego has areas of weakness that could open the way to sudden disorganisation, for example, death of the father, aggravation of conflicts with her husband, etc. For the time being, in the absence of medical information, psychosomatic risk is low to moderate.

The medical file

Let's take a look at the medical record and the somatic risk. Béatrice consults in October 1991 for a large left-breast tumour that is treated with first-line chemotherapy and radiotherapy. Then she refuses the proposed mastectomy but accepts complementary brachytherapy. Five years later, in July 1996, a cutaneous recurrence treated by hormonotherapy appears. As markers continue to increase, eight-month chemotherapy is prescribed. In October 1997, she accepted a mastectomy-reconstruction by large dorsal. In June 2002, she receives tamoxifen hormone therapy, then two other drugs; despite everything, permeation nodules appear.

Since then she has been on arimidex and tamoxifen. In August 2003, the nodules appear to be under control but remain present and visible. In February 2005, the are nodules still stable. There is no further spread. In December 2008 she is still being treated, and the many side effects are starting to affect her life. A therapeutic break for a month is then attempted, but this is difficult psychologically and there is no clinical improvement, contrary to the initial expectation. The nodules have not changed but they persist and are visible, and therefore anxiety-inducing, particularly as the serum markers are slowly rising.

Medical prognosis and psychosomatic prognosis

Béatrice is a patient who observes but who asks explanations of the doctors, often in a demanding, and even argumentative, way. Béatrice wants to understand and actively participate in all decisions. For doctors, the medical prognosis is not good. Personally, and paradoxically, I disagree with the medical prognosis because I think that Béatrice has mental capabilities to defend herself against the breast cancer, abilities that have never been evaluated by the doctors at any point over the last eight years.

They know nothing about her mental defences and the capacities of her spirit! They are therefore always pessimistic! Hence, there are many recommendations for chemotherapy. Doctors do not understand her life drive and her capacity for resistance: they never question her!

In subsequent sessions, Béatrice talks about her childhood and describes herself as a tomboy, a happy but rebellious child. For her, her mother was a submissive, stifled, impersonal, depressed woman who looked after the household and was silent. She makes excuses for her mother by saying that she had a very difficult childhood. As for her father, she has always clashed with him, but they love each other very much. He himself lost his father at six years old and a sister at eighteen years old, of tuberculosis. The relationship with the father, which I followed until his death, is affectionate and close. She loves her father very much. The oedipal conflict was present. Béatrice is the second child of a family of three. Her older brother lives as a drop-out in the Larzac. As for her sister, their relationship seems distant, but Béatrice knows she can count on her in the event of difficulties, something that she proved by accompanying Béatrice to all her chemotherapy sessions. The two women are both close and distant. Béatrice did only one year of graduate school, and she regrets not having pursued her studies, but she is catching up by taking classes at the Sorbonne.

The imaginary dimension and Béatrice's beliefs

Béatrice has a spiritual approach to research and supports herself with alternative medicine. She feels comfortable in nature, cultivates a garden, and meditates in the moonlight or at sunset. During the therapy, over many years, we build a relationship that allows me to encourage her in her relationship with her reflexologist, with whom she meets often. Having read numerous scientific studies on touch and body massage, I suggested that she ask her reflexologist to massage her feet for more than twenty minutes rather just a few. I noted in a major epidemiological study that a massage lasting more than twenty minutes activates the function and expression of certain genes that strengthen the heart and the immune system. I think it is worth trying. Surprisingly, when the markers are high, this twenty-minute foot massage allowed her, within a few days, to fulfil the biological conditions necessary to take up chemotherapy! Extensive epidemiological studies would be required to understand these mysterious somatic mechanisms.

In addition, Béatrice had a mystical relationship with her garden and the trees in her garden. So, I tried, with her, to act on her psychosomatic economy (to restore her energy); I once again suggested going to the garden and mentally soliciting the energy of the trees by placing her hands on the trunks. She was very comfortable with this particular activity and it seemed to have some effect! All this is far from being able to be confirmed scientifically, but it must be understood that my suggestions did appear to cause a rise in the level of mental defences, with, as far as I could tell, meaningful consequences for the immune system, which was confirmed by the significant drop in somatic markers. I used the same techniques of traditional therapies with patients from North Africa and sub-Saharan Africa: acting on beliefs through symbolic acts.

Béatrice was married at the age of twenty-three to a man who, like her, had received a strict education with much prejudice around sexuality. Coming from an unhappy background, she thought she could help him. But he remained introverted and without friends. She describes their relationship as warm and supportive, yet she laments that he sees her more as a mother. She did not have children, due to an unexplained fertility problem. Her husband refused to investigate this and opposed adoption. This remained very painful for Béatrice since, she says, "the breast represents motherhood." Even though there was no biological analysis to understand this problem of infertility, we can at least hypothesise about it: she grew up like a tomboy, and the journey towards the oedipal conflict was first worked out in rivalry with the father, then, gradually, with the progress of the analytic therapy, in a progressive investment of the feminine dimension. We must understand that the main problem is the psychic investment in the body to be able to access feminine psychic identity. For her, the breast was the symbol of breast-feeding, which, unfortunately, was something that could not be realised!

Summary of issues and questions about the strength of mental functioning

I remember that Béatrice, before her cancer, was very invested in her work. It was a rewarding activity; she was hyperactive and had excellent relationships with her colleagues and her managers. She was the victim of significant professional stress due to the risk of being dismissed, and therefore at financial risk, which disrupted her psychic balance and, eventually, her somatic balance. Her ability to invest in the world enabled her to continue her life by enrolling in art history courses in the Sorbonne; she then enrolled in gymnastics classes. Throughout her therapy, Béatrice complained of arm lymphoedema and multiple pains. As of 2009, the side effects of heavy, aggressive treatments became more difficult to live with. In terms of somatic symptoms, I must add the mourning of her mother in 2005, with sequelae that we treated in therapy to overcome this traumatic event. As for her father, threatened with respiratory failure and heart problems, I can say that she supported him emotionally and courageously until his death.

The side effects of her hormone therapy always worried me, and they started to be very harmful. According to her gynaecologist, this treatment is limited because permeation nodules do not regress and the markers slowly rise. I struggled alongside Béatrice for years in her resistance to the various effects of chemotherapy. It is with sadness, at the end of this presentation, that I must announce that Béatrice died of the chemotherapy that her body could not cope with. Her death, which I did not anticipate, deeply affected me and I wondered for a long time about the fact that her oncologist had not consulted me so that together we could have evaluated the psychic and somatic resistance abilities of my dear patient.

This clinical example encourages us to reflect on the global nature of psychosomatic unity: the strength of her mental defences allowed Béatrice to engage in a survival strategy, but the body no longer had any resistance and death followed.

A psychosomatist must be able to cope with the death of his patients by understanding that a process of mourning ensues and that he must analyse it in order to accept the death.

Géraldine: a rational fighter

In 2011, I had a first interview with Géraldine, then aged forty-six; she had been referred to me for breast cancer. I will first present the various interviews I had with her over the ensuing five years by inserting the questions that came to my mind as our relationship unfolded, and then I will present an elaboration of the case indicating the diagnosis that I propose with reference to the new integrative psychosomatics nosography (see Appendix 2).

Géraldine tells me immediately: "I did not feel sick, neither in my head nor in my body; I am completely wrapped up." What does she mean by that? Does she want to tell me that she did not feel any damage to her body? Is she really protected, as she says? If she is right, she has emotional support to resist the disease. "Now I have to endure things that are difficult to manage." Géraldine is perhaps going through a moment in her life that we must explore together. What are these difficult things?

For ten years, she says, "I had a nodule in the left breast; I had an ultrasound, nothing more. Whenever there was a blow in my life, I felt a pain, a kind of burning at the top of the nodule; it was in June, July 2010." Géraldine is not the first patient who has shared with me her bodily feelings following difficult life events. So, there is sensory communication that she can access by being able to suggest an interpretation.

> I lived with my daughter's father for fifteen years and left a little over ten years ago. I lived for three and a half years with one person; it was an impossible relationship, it had to be stopped. We separated; it was the greatest pain of my life. I lost five pounds in ten days; I face up to everything, all alone. I was working for an international transport company that closed at the same time. It was a difficult period. I have graduate degrees and so I have a high level of qualifications.

Géraldine tells me about her life and the traumatic events accompanying it; unlike her first statement, she confirms that she "faces everything, all alone". What appears very clearly is the way the psychic apparatus overflows, unable to cope with the very high quantum of excitations assaulting the patient.

Géraldine then goes on to talk about her family relationships, first with her sister and her brothers, then with her parents.

> In 2008 I helped my little sister who is several years younger than me and who called for me to be at her side; but she fled to

the police and asked to be interned. I became the legal representative of my sister on the recommendation of her psychiatrist;
I have a maternal role to her. I have a brother a little younger
than me and another brother who is ten years younger. I made a
suicide attempt two years after my departure from my parents'
home; they did not understand that I see psychiatrists. From the
summer of 2008, my parents did not want to see me again. I felt
like an orphan. I got my first job in Paris a year later; that's when
I sold my apartment to pay for my studies. I had known my
daughter's father since the age of eighteen; I collapsed because
my daughter's father cut off the financial support. There was no
more money in the accounts; in truth I had been stolen from for
eight years.

Géraldine continues the story, which focuses mainly on personal and
family relationships. She becomes the legal guardian of her sister, and
she is abandoned by her parents. Then she must deal with a dramatic
financial situation created by her ex-husband. It is obvious that the
accumulation of non-mentalized dramatic situations cannot but have a
disastrous effect on somatic functioning.

In the summer of 2009, I prepared a procedure for him to pay
me a pension; my daughter wanted to live in Paris. She found a
file against me in her father's house; I did not have a home and
insufficient salary to get one. My daughter is attending an excellent high school. During the summer of 2009, I had a fixed-term
contract in a real estate agency. I did not find work. I hope to
have an interview in a company.

Géraldine demonstrates perseverance and a fighting spirit; it is important to understand the origin of this resilience.

I felt the first pain in April of the following year after opening
the envelope that came from the courts; it was money for my
daughter's education. I remained friends with my stepfather.
At the end of June 2010, there was still uncertainty about where
to live; at that time, I received a very large tax adjustment and it
was very shocking for me. I also had to face the hostility of my

husband's new partner. I felt a burning in the breast, and I saw a gynaecologist who thought it was nothing, that it was benign. I thought there was something. So, I had a biopsy and at the end of October 2010, I had results. I meet again with my doctor who tells me about a serious illness; she does not pronounce the word cancer, she says, "That little thing, you have to have it off." So, I made an appointment at the breast clinic, and the surgeon answered all my questions; what he said corresponded to what I had expected. I was operated on in November and the sentinel lymph nodes were not affected.

It is important to listen to patients; Géraldine has a great capacity for sensory perception and her gynaecologist did not listen. It is important that we train our doctors better to listen to their patients. In addition, her gynaecologist was not prepared for the announcement of cancer.

Thanks to this operation, everything was positive; I turned a page and got in touch with my parents. You know, people looking at you make you sick. I am someone who veils her face; I am an eternal optimist, polarised by my professional success. My father was a political refugee, and he destroyed his family; I am not afraid of him. As for my mother, she tested teaching methods in primary school; at the age of four, five, I did not know how to do maths and I had reading problems; I was left-handed and they wanted me to retake a year to make me right-handed! I was a committed left-hander. The teacher did not want me to retake the year and this is the time of the first break with my mother. I came to my senses at the age of twenty-five; I really like human relations. My best friend was my dog who for ten years was my companion.

Géraldine reveals here the roots of her capacity for mental resistance: confronted with a very early conflict concerning the use of the left hand, thanks to her teacher she was able to triumph over a conflict with her mother. She also tells me about her opposition to a father who, she says, destroyed her family. Everything is based on a narcissism that has been reinforced over the years. Without this dimension, she would not have survived. Finally, it is important to note the role of her dog that supported her for ten years. This is not the first time I have encountered the way in which a dog can offer psychic support to its owner. Thanks to her teacher, Géraldine chose the path of cognitive and intellectual development, which allowed her to mature and at the same time constituted a defence system known as "defensive intellectualisation".

"It was at the end of 1998 that I had my first love relationship; I have a network of friends. I do not have a spiritual life, I am agnostic. I breastfed my daughter for six months." Géraldine finishes this first interview by informing me that she has support from a network of friends, but that she has no spiritual resources. When talking to me about feeding her daughter, she wanted to give me the image of a good mother. I remembered this image when asking questions about Géraldine's relationship with her own mother.

I meet Géraldine a year later; she is still having difficulties finding work.

> I thought I had found a stable position with a perfumer, but it did not work. I was not in the right place, and it was a bogus job based on a lie. I have no desire at all for that world, I am caring; I also worked for a sculptor voluntarily. I had a row with the director. I am now working for myself, but in a month I will no longer have unemployment benefits! I know the president of an association who could help me.

I say that she is very brave. Géraldine reveals here her abilities of resistance and perseverance.

> I refuse to be abused; all these corporate restructurings are violent and decided upon following mergers; I have a lot of experience of the big industrial groups in which I worked. After my breast cancer surgery, I called my father and mother. My mother called me every morning so as to feel less guilty; my father never called me. Today, I feel like an orphan; it does not hurt me. No more relationships, neither words nor gestures, I will manage. I rented a small apartment, and my daughter left to continue her studies abroad. Coming back to the subject of the behaviour of my parents, I can say that nobody was there for me.

That's the truth, Géraldine cannot count on either her father or her mother; she is alone.

> I expected compensation from the industrial tribunals, but nothing yet. To defend myself, I have an instinctual side; I can still trust. It's mostly men who have betrayed me. With my daughter's father, we lived very well, but I knew that I did not want to make my life with him. With my new relationship, at Easter 2011, I moved away, but after the summer, at the time of his birthday, I got back together with him. In human relations, time is the best of allies. This is the first time I have been attached to someone; apparently, I have changed. My daughter told me, "There is something going on." I think that with this man it was not possible to say goodbye. This is the first time I have felt such a feeling; as for him, he had been betrayed by women.

Géraldine's ordeals helped her grow; she came out of her isolation and started to establish an object relationship. However, she reveals to me that she has great difficulty in establishing a relationship with men, and she chose an emotional relationship with a man who is her mirror since he himself has difficulties in his relations with women!

> I had breast surgery and I had radiation therapy for two and a half months; there is a check every six months. I saw the surgeon and my gynaecologist. The next step will be the mammogram next May or June. All this changed the order of my priorities. In truth, I felt the disease coming and as soon as I saw the surgeon everything was very fast. He was the first to say the word "cancer" by answering all my questions. I never felt sick either in my body or in my head. In my case, what helps me is that I did not have a religious education. I have not been educated with the notion of suffering. As for the disease, for me it was like an axe. Unfair, undeserving, and very violent. At that point I said to myself: everything is over.

Cancer has flicked a particular switch. The disease has affected her body and, in some way, has changed her relationship to the world. I can note two important developments: a change in the relationship with the other and the awareness of a body that is not yet psyche but could become so in the context of psychotherapy. For the moment everything rests on her redeeming narcissism.

> This cancer gave me a new vision of life; my priorities are no longer in the same order. For me, the body is a tool because I had a nice body and I have always been aware of it. Sex does not interest me; I need to be seduced by an image. I want to age well. I pay attention to my body. I really admire some artists who take care of their bodies.

These statements confirm the narcissistic investment in the body and her psychosexual immaturity because the genital dimension has not yet been developed. "I am convinced that this disease has been sent to me; I've met people who spoke to me about this and I am convinced that my maternal grandfather protects me." At the end of this session, Géraldine suddenly tells me of archaic beliefs that support her psyche. Her maternal grandfather protects her unconsciously and consciously. The appearance of this figure is for me reassuring because I used to work with patients from African and Asian cultures in which one is protected by the way in which beliefs in the existence of ancestors influence contemporary life. "As a child," she says, "I was an observer; now I'm waiting for it all to happen."

The third meeting is when I see Géraldine four years later as part of my ongoing breast cancer research. She talks to me, first, about her work:

> I have a job that involves food and I have a lot of contacts that will enable me to change jobs. I am exploited and I want my salary doubled. I am now working in a cooperative, in health insurance. I am not paid for my real skill. I am worried and at times it annoys me a little. The man I met four years ago has become a very close friend; it's a choice. I am a single person and now it is he who is sick; I must respect his choice. I feel able to be with him, but I cannot put myself in his place. At present, I have a recurrence of cancer, and I was operated on by another surgeon. I again felt a burning sensation that I associate with difficult times. I have to give up, to accept that I cannot live with this man. In addition,

> I was between jobs, and I was faced with the search for a new job. I am well, I am happy, there is, in the depths of me, a redoubling of effort, an alertness that does not show itself, that does not go inside. In addition, I have to move house again, and there, it's like everything is reassembled, all the past is back. I was not ready, fed up, time flies, I asked for my breast to be removed, the breast that is being rebuilt. There is no metastasis.

In a few sentences, Géraldine tells me about the recurrence of breast cancer caused by life events that are difficult to mentalize: job difficulties, a move that reactivates the pain of the past, and, finally, an attack on the body, the mastectomy. We must note here the sensory perception of the modification of the body. "The oncologist advised a preventative chemo and I fought to keep my hair. I am a woman of action."

We can see, throughout our interviews, that Géraldine distanced herself from her feelings; for me, it is more a repression of feelings rather than an absence of feelings, of emotions; that is, alexithymia. This is the narcissistic dimension to a Géraldine who does not want to be weak in front of me; she is and will always remain a fighter.

> I have been taking an anti-cancer drug for two months. I have advanced in the last five years. I am no longer in denial; I avoided being sick, I did not feel sick. For the breast reconstruction, I've paid attention to the most aesthetic result possible. In my work for the insurance company, I've developed various aspects and I've given the boss a year to increase my salary. I have a good relationship with him and I have a good relationship with my doctors. I got back in touch with my brother and met my sister-in-law; I now manage to maintain emotional ties. In fact, if I'd had a family, I would not have cancer. Today, I speak.

I was very happy to have met Géraldine.

Some psychosomatic reflections

Géraldine has a psychic functioning of a narcissistic nature. The self, the first psychosomatic structure of a human being, is the predominant nucleus. She therefore has a very fragile personality because the process of maturation stopped very early in her development. Her mental defence is defensive intellectualisation. She has strongly invested in the intellectual processes that are revealed by her desire for professional success and the acquisition of diplomas. All her speech is dominated by intellectuality: there is poor imagination and little or no associative capacity. Unconscious processes create significant breaks in communication. In a relationship with a mother who has remained a pre-object for her, Géraldine has built important mental defences based on primary narcissism; she is fixed in a relation to a cleaved maternal object, namely the bad mother and the good mother. The bad-mother side was strengthened because her mother wanted her to become right-handed. It seems to me that this constraint allowed Géraldine to preserve what Dr René Árpád Spitz called the "coenesthetic organisation", namely the sensorimotor abilities at the beginning of life; abilities that eventually become unconscious. This sensory sensitivity allowed her to detect the symptoms of breast cancer well in advance. She appears to be affirming her femininity, but her inability to invest an object relation is detrimental to the establishment of deep relationships with an object. Her first husband had the role of maternal support. She is stuck in a romantic teenage position, again revealing the difficulty of integrating sexual urges. The feminine psychic identity has never developed, and the patient remains fixed in a narcissistic position with a primary, and not a secondary, masochistic nucleus.

In conclusion, there is a fragile mental apparatus, overwhelmed by any traumatic event, and a low capacity for elaboration. She remains on a narcissistic base to protect herself from what endangers the self because it is not only the guarantor of the integrity of the psychosomatic unity but also the place of disorganisation with no going back, that is to say, it is the threat of the appearance of a narcissism of death. She sought escape from maternal deprivation in an investment of knowledge. Indeed, she is only slightly older than her brother. The two children who followed her birth have significant mental disorders, revealing maternal deficiencies.

Second examination

The illness, which was initially denied, seems to have influenced the patient's perceptions. It has changed the priorities of her life; for the first time, she has a romantic relationship even though her narcissism prevents her from having an object relationship. The other begins to have an independent existence; she comes out of her solipsism. The ego of the patient changes slowly in an objectal direction, of a maternal type (the search for affection). My hypothesis is that the process of psychic maturation restarted thanks to the modification of the body of which she became aware; it was her body that helped her.

Géraldine has gone through hard times in the professional field and overcome them. She is currently involved in the takeover of businesses with the help of a pensioners' association, a lawyer, and an accountant. The future seems a little more certain but is accompanied by considerable risks. She is not alone though. I would say that the "narcissism of life" supports her, but that the irregularities of mental functioning are always present. She is a fighter.

Third examination

Géraldine is in the process of professional retraining, and she has found a position where she considers that she is not paid well enough for her level of true competency. The man she met four years ago has become a very close friend.

It's a choice she says: once again, looking for the affection of the object, genital sexuality still does not exist. She is single. "He's the one who's sick and I feel able to be with him, but I cannot put myself in his place," she says. She tells me she has a recurrence of the cancer and that she has been operated on by her first surgeon's colleague. Two years ago, she again felt the burning in her body, following a significant event: she realised that she could not live with the man who was her companion. She was unemployed, with anxiety about her job seeking. Overwhelmed by excitations following on from rapid disorganisation, the cancer returned.

"I'm fine, I'm happy inside me, like a kind of duplication." In addition to this problem of separation, there was the move and all her past being reactivated. Everything got worse in the summer of 2013. A year later, the cancer recurred: it was a moment of exhaustion. She therefore asked for the removal of a breast and it is being reconstructed. There are no metastases; the oncologist has advised preventive chemotherapy.

Psychic functioning is more stable, moving towards a return to equilibrium. It is a question of "normopathy", as described by Joyce

McDougall (1978), dominated by behaviour, without itself being a behavioural neurosis.

Diagnosis

On the axis of self-conservation, there are narcissistic personality disorders, and normopathy in relation to a maternal pre-object; the transfer neurosis is partly developed.

I establish, following investigation, the evaluation of the psychosomatic risk. The subject is at medium risk: the defence ability is in a defensive intellectualisation mode, and can give way quickly to traumatic events related to changes in the environment. However, we can count on the strength of primary narcissism. Due to the immaturity of mental defences, the patient is deprived of adaptability, whatever the nature of the environment. If the environment is stable, it will have the ability to resist. The concern is about the future environment and her vulnerability; therefore, I reserve my prognosis for the future. During the second examination, I find that Géraldine resists and is still on the side of life: there is a partner, optimism about a professional project, and a return to a family history that is stabilising. The psychosomatic risks decrease considerably. I am more optimistic.

Laura: a life of pain

I met Laura two years before I left my consultation at the Pitié-Salpêtrière Hospital. Laura was sixty-eight years old and she told me a lot about her painful life from the age of twelve. When dealing with chronic pain in the life of a human being, it is always important to ask about the role of pain in the psychosomatic balance? The second question is always: what can a psychosomatist do for such patients? Other than by medical prescription, how can we help them?

The story of Laura's life will allow me to elaborate hypotheses to better understand the psychodynamics of her personality. Laura is a woman of exceptional intelligence who has held very high public office. She describes several important phases of her life; these four phases are qualified by significant upheavals.

First phase: twelve to twenty years of age

"At twelve," she tells me, "a doctor discovered significant scoliosis." Laura is standing in front of me in my consulting office and it seems that there is something wrapped around her upper body to keep it upright. I think she is used to wearing a type of corset; she sits in a chair in front of me, very comfortably. As a result of her initial diagnosis, Laura was admitted to the hospital for sick children and underwent, as she specifies, barbaric treatments, which her mother appeared to be indifferent to. One can immediately think about her age with this first diagnosis, which was twelve; a critical age when they are changes occurring in the body and the girl is being transformed into a teenager moving into the genital phase of the development. We immediately understand that this treatment halted the process of the development of psychosexual maturation. Laura has remained stuck in this period and in a relationship with a mother whose emotional characteristics will gradually make themselves known in the story.

She describes three kinds of "barbaric" treatment: the "torture of the gallows" ("the name used by therapists", she says): suspended pulleys and ropes, with a leather halter. This technique results in separating the vertebrae and weakening the spinal column. When you are "suspended" there is a feeling like having your head crushed by a life. She does not say anything to her mother, who never accompanies her, even though she was only twelve years old! The second torture is that of the "espalier": "back to the wall, suspended by the hands to a horizontal bar, while two cushions are placed at the location of my dorsal and lumber gibbosities. This has the effect of making any impact very painful." The third torture is that of restraint, twenty-four hours a day:

> I sleep in a plaster shell, they wrap me up like a mummy because I tend to sleep on my side; during the day, I wear an orthopaedic corset made of pink leather with eighteen iron bands and leather rings that pull the arms back and are crossed at the back. This gives you a totally stiff outline and limits the movements of the hands.

To all these techniques of straightening the spine are added prohibitions: absolutely no sport, gymnastics, running, jumping. "In the schoolyard,

I am invisible, I do not play any games and I work: I do not appear on any class photo from the eighth grade till the end of school."

How did Laura experience these traumatic treatments? She says she attributes the worsening of her scoliosis, up to the age of twenty, to these barbaric treatments. "Coming out of Necker's sessions, I rush to the bakery opposite and devour enormous cakes. I put on 20 to 30 pounds." Laura is still young and has the resources to make up for her pain and frustrations by eating cake, which is positive in a way, but certainly with the risk of becoming overweight. It is important to be very careful in our assessments. A human being must be able to have a little fun in her life.

Laura continues and explains how she has managed to develop thanks to great intelligence and a huge capacity for intellectual work.

> I am very bright in my studies. My mother lugs me around to
> like a scholarly monkey with my report cards, showing them off
> to the whole family. I feel like a circus freak. I work non-stop,
> including holidays. It's the only way to get my parents' attention
> and win their love.

This is the motivation: to be loved by one's father and mother. But what are her parents and who are they? The answer to this question will allow us to understand the search for pain.

Second phase

When she was aged nineteen, her father died suddenly, of a brain tumour, at age fifty, during an operation. In the period of mourning for the father, her two-year-old sister began to show disturbing signs of mental imbalance and was detained in the Saint-Anne hospital with a diagnosis of schizophrenia. Three months later, her mother was detained for manic depressive psychosis and began a period of thirty-two years of psychiatric follow-up with periods of detainment and remission. Financial problems appear: in twenty years the mother spends the family fortune and the family is ruined. What to do then when you are twenty years old?

> I find myself alone with an eighty-five-year-old grandmother
> and a maid who cannot read or write. I work full-time during

the day to pay for my father's debts and support the family. And at night, I continue my studies. I break my "shell" with hammers, and I burn my corset in the kitchen: it is in 1968. I meet my future husband on the barricades. I have children, which the doctors have advised me against. I lost 14 pounds during my first pregnancy and 14 pounds in the second. There is not a single degree of new back curvature. I became a beautiful young woman, and I am very surprised by my success with men, which annoys my husband who used to make fun of my body.

What happened and how to interpret the changes? The events of 1968 profoundly altered the social pressure on sexual prohibition. Laura greatly benefited to the extent that the parental prohibitions disappeared, which allowed the libido to pursue its direction, resulting in an investment of the body and the authorisation to have a sex life of a genital nature. Social liberation allowed her to marry and have two children. But what has happened to the pain? From the age of twenty to the age of forty, Laura has put all her energy into sport and work, keeping the pain away. Has the disease disappeared? This is what we will examine carefully.

From twenty to forty years old, it is an adult period of denial. I do not care. I cross out my scoliosis and I pretend I don't have anything. I play sports, dance, cycle, I work a lot. I am very active, I create a dozen associations, including a local newspaper, a free radio, and cooperatives.

Third critical phase

But, contrary to what Laura says, at the age of thirty-two, there is a new earthquake!

I celebrate my ten years of marriage with my husband. We go to see a Bergman film, *The Egg and the Snake*, about the destruction of a couple in Nazi Germany. During the screening, seeing a close-up of the male character behind the bars of his bed, I am seized with an unspeakable anguish: I start screaming, rolling on the floor. I am taken to the emergency department and I begin eleven years of hell, with anxiety attacks that crash down on top of me without my understanding why and whose frequency increases dramatically: I become totally claustrophobic. My life becomes impossible, I cannot stand lifts, tunnels, queues in shops, public transport, cinemas, restaurants, subways, the tube, the overground. At no time do I stop working. I refuse any medication (given the family history), I am in permanent suffering: apart from crises, I remain on the alert, in fear of what comes next. I take up NLP therapy for seven years and then have seven years of psychoanalysis.

Why does Laura feel threatened and what are the sequences of Bergman's film that reactivated a deep sense of threat?

Berlin, in 1923, a pack of cigarettes costs 4 billion marks. It's galloping inflation, unemployment, misery, and despair. Amid the chaos, Abel Rosenberg feels triply alienated as he is Jewish, American, and unemployed. While he gets lost in alcohol, Abel discovers the body of his brother who has shot himself in the mouth. Questioned by the police, he has the sense that he is suspected of several murders that have been perpetrated in the neighbourhood. He takes refuge with Manuela, the former companion of his brother, who performs in a number of low-life cabarets. Together, they live out a perverse relationship and go about in fear, threatened by an unspeakable evil that "like a snake's egg, reveals, through its thin shell, the form of a perfect reptile". The film's title refers to a tirade by Brutus in Shakespeare's *Julius Caesar*: "And therefore think him as a snake's egg/Which hatched, would as his kind grow mischievous,/And kill him in the shell."

The death threat: destiny of father and mother

It is my hypothesis that this film has reactivated the death of her father for whom the mourning has never been completed, and the traumatic fate of her bi-polar mother undergoing constant internment and squandering the family fortune. Laura explains it very well: "This is a film about the destruction of a couple!" Anxiety invades her life.

Laura's life continues, and she explains that because of her mental decompensation, she has lived as a single person, with her children in shared custody. Then she meets a violent man and becomes a beaten and humiliated woman, to the point of being incapable of separating from him. She ends up escaping this man's unbearable brutality. To avoid meeting him at their shared place of work, she invests all her energy in a postgraduate degree, spending part of her nights studying. She is successful; she graduates from her class and is offered a position in the office of the Prime Minister.

Psychopathology of pain

We now better understand Laura's psychopathology and its relation to pain. What does pain represent? Pain is a bad internalised object; her entire history, from the first years of life, reflects a pre-object relationship with a mother who rejects her and who persecutes her. To obtain the love of this mother, and her father, she has strongly invested in the intellectual dimension. By becoming a good student, she imagined that she could obtain the love of her parents. She did get it, but in an internalised and sadistic way. Since the pre-object was internalised in a sadistic form, the pain took over and replaced it. Laura can only live without pain if, on the therapeutic level, a global object that include both characteristics (good and bad) is not internalised. Without pain, Laura cannot continue her life. We can now understand her relationship with a body that persecutes her and absorbs all external and internal tensions. The body suffers but protects her. The circle is complete.

The last phases

Laura's story continues, and she recounts the traumas of her life. In 1986, aged thirty-nine, she meets, on the anniversary of the death of her father, a man she falls madly in love; this man looks amazing to her, and she abandons everything to live with him. She gets pregnant the following year and has an ectopic pregnancy with internal bleeding. A huge depression follows and the curvature of her spine gets worse. She enters a period of terrible anxiety attacks and resumes psychoanalysis. In 1997, her mother dies and she joins a ministerial cabinet, in which she invests heavily; it sets up programmes for youth employment. "I work night and day, I leave work at 1 or 2 am, I sleep at the hotel across the street … I sometimes spend a whole week without going home." She manages to create tens of thousands of jobs; she participates in three other ministerial cabinets. She goes through another dramatic period. As she puts it, "I am entering a period of tremendous moral persecution." She invests her energy once more in her battle to save jobs.

> In the meantime, my health has become much worse. I have my menopause, I suffer terribly from my back, I walk bent forward. I have a serious respiratory attack, fortunately, a few meters away from a pneumology department where I'm put under an oxygen tent. Then a real obstacle course begins. I have X-rays. I cannot believe it. The balance sheet has become catastrophic. I'm making myself extremely ill. I'm going to see the greatest French spine surgeons. They all refuse to operate. Reason: a transplant of the spine happens in two stages: a lung is blocked to graft a rib, and likewise on the other side. But this involves huge risk for a surgeon and no insurance will cover it. Six months later, I try to get up, I howl: my hip bangs on my chest. My rib cage is so crushed that it causes osteolysis: in the morning I can walk with two canes, in the afternoon, I am bedridden. I cannot sit down anymore, can no longer move my left leg.

Laura can no longer stand: she falls forward and she is forced to lean against something to stand. She no longer has any balance, which refers, it is still my hypothesis, to maternal deprivation since her mother never held or supported her. How can we stand upright if our mother has not support us? And then, if the spine does not support us? She goes to see the final surgeon on her list, who sets three goals: lose 10 kilograms, regain verticality, and regain vital lung capacity. To get through this period, Laura uses a behavioural therapist who supports her in her aims. She is heroic, and the surgeon agrees to operate. She survives in a hostile environment. In 2005, she underwent an almost total transplant of the spine: seventeen vertebrae. These are extreme measures that she is taking. After the operation, she is literally "abandoned" in a nursing home, without a permanent doctor.

She is injected with massive doses of drugs containing morphine, benzodiazepines, and analgesics.

In this emotional desert, she is saved by a friend who calls her every day. We create a method that uses the happy memories of the music of my grandmother pianist and my uncle violinist whose music comforted me in my childhood and I visualise, with each piece that I remember internally, the dissolution of the crystals of my inner ear. We manage to remove any symptoms in a month and a half. She has bone pain and unbearable bone-marrow burns. Moreover, she is completely isolated emotionally from her family. In 2006, she finally returns home, where life is difficult because she cannot go upstairs and has to live on the ground floor. To finance the adaption of her house, she has the extraordinary idea of rewriting theses for PhD students in difficulty. She is very successful in this area because she is a very talented person. Life is always totally dramatic, but she is always able to find solutions. I admire this ability a lot.

A few years later, she has pain again and is diagnosed with depression, which is not surprising because she is using a lot of vital energy. In addition, she must undergo a new operation to straighten her spine. She has a drug addiction crisis and decides to wean herself off all the painkillers, which causes her to have serious anxiety attacks. One day, during a short walk on a deserted path, she loses all control of her legs. She calls for help: there is no one, and she has no mobile phone. Almost paralysed, it takes more than an hour and a half to return home. To help with her coming off the medication, she participates in a therapy group and succeeds in stopping taking the painkillers. It takes two and a half years to put an end to this ordeal. She can return to work at the ministry, but she is hidden away. The bone and muscle pains are so strong that she holds out for only eight months without any medicine. She is forced to resume treatment. She suffers from unbearable anxiety attacks that prevent her, at times, from driving, to attend meetings, to go outside. She takes Lexomil in moderate doses.

The meeting with Laura

When I met Laura, and considering the archaic dimensions of her personality, I took her into follow-up therapy and referred her to a colleague, a body therapist, to help her establish psychic connections with her body, and no longer just sensory-motor links unattached to thought. At the same time, she had a homeopathic follow-up, auriculotherapy, and sophrology. We must understand here that Laura faced a quantum of excitations at such a pitch that required all these various therapies to fulfil the role of a weekly protective shield. Even so, this did not prevent very painful, frequent crises of several kinds, which required increased does of Lexomil, or even being taking into emergency care or for oxygenation. Laura described the return of the sensations she experienced when she was diagnosed with scoliosis at the age of twelve.

Some thoughts

The return of those sensations tells us that a psychic regression is at work and that the set of problems for which she has been followed therapeutically for many years has still not been resolved. We are faced with a patient totally dominated by cognitive-rational thinking, and by the primary narcissism[8] which has ensured the continuity of life until now. The integration of a persecutory object was made through body pain. This pain has never been mainstreamed and the primary object relationship could not be developed through the internalisation process.

What should be done? Is it possible to analyse the extremely solid defence system developed over more than fifty years, and get it to evolve? What can be done to help Laura? There are two possible strategies: one is to build psychosomatic unity in the body through psychocorporal therapy, and that is what I recommended; at the same time, to undertake a weekly supportive therapy to ensure the role of excitatory shields to gradually replace psychotropic drugs, and especially to start developing the basis of a solid psychic system. One could, from the support therapy, develop, whatever the age of the patient, an attachment relationship leading to the construction of an object that could be internalised and safeguard the patient by modifying her defence system.

---

[8] In primary narcissism, the child invests all his psychic energy (the libido) on himself; this first investment can assure his survival in the event of trauma.

This second part was not possible because the administration of the hospital had adopted a new policy and ended my consultation after twenty-one years of working with patients! The trauma-related death anxiety has accompanied Laura all her life and only the analysis of grief and trauma would have finally allowed her to end it.

CHAPTER 4

Psychosomatic enigmas

The psychosomatic consultation at the hospital can sometimes become strange because we must deal with patients without a diagnosis. The doctor or myself are unable to establish a diagnosis, *a fortiori* a treatment, or even the direction of the cure. We are in the dark, and I would like to present a few cases to illustrate my point.

Sandrine: beyond nephrological disorders, a desperate patient

"Sandrine, you are now healed!" Sandrine was referred to me by a colleague in the nephrology department; my colleague simply told her, "You are now healed!" This was the beginning of the medical wanderings of my patient. At first, she had sought the support of her first doctor and as she considered that the treatment was successful, there was nothing more to be done. In desperation, the nephologist sent this patient to me, thinking that maybe I could do something for her. I wondered at length about the use of the term "cure". Can a doctor tell a patient that he or she is cured? How is that done?

I receive Sandrine, who begins to summarise the letter she wrote to her GP and describes all the troubles she has suffered since she was "cured". She writes that she wants to inform her doctor of her condition since the last visit: after her visit to the emergency department in December, she was again very affected throughout the weekend. She describes with great precision the picture of her symptoms: tremors, chills, stress in the chest, palpitations, burns and chest pain, spinal pain, great difficulty breathing even taking a few steps, shortness of breath, headache, the sensation of almost permanent suffocation, great exhaustion. And in addition: "Obviously under these conditions, a small meal stifles me."

She rests completely during the Sunday and, on Monday evening, the same kind of discomfort, even if the tachycardia is now more limited. She still feels the pulsing in her head that has been present since March. As for post-meal discomfort and choking, that appeared in March, April, and May. Yesterday and today, she has less trouble, so she stand up a little easier! In the best of cases, she has severe pain all over the left side (lumbar, abdomen) and, in any case, severe pain in the shins and ankles, seriously interfering with her ability to function, "if any still remains!" she adds. In the evening, there is still burning in the lower body and pain diffusing into the lower limbs and thorax, with tremors and chills.

The urine test strip is still positive for leukocytes and the urine is dark yellow and cloudy. And yet the latest CBEU (cytobacteriological examination of urine) has an insignificant result according to her doctor, which annoys Sandrine because she cannot bear any disagreement around his observations. She continues, "I went under the bar of 52 kilos now. And the periods when I can carry out some activities, even locked up, are more and more rare. I did the MIBG scan yesterday and today. The doctor must make his report (*a priori* negative, to be confirmed)." The doctor, not knowing what to say to such a patient, tells her that it is difficult to appreciate certain images because she is thin. She must meet her cardiologist and does not believe that she can make the effort to take the stress test. She will keep her general practitioner informed; she has extreme difficulties in moving and she is weakened as a result of the excessive duration of this situation. She concluded her letter by hoping that her doctor can appreciate the seriousness of her condition and will come up with a quick solution that is adapted to the help of the specialists she must consult, without waiting until she has to go back to the emergency room, or be permanently bedridden!

The role of the disease and the medical enigma

As soon as Sandrine was "cured", her doctor, without noticing it, suppressed the somatic disorder that absorbed all sensory and motor stimuli. In fact, the disease had played a considerable balancing role. As soon as she was cured, all the excitations coming from her family and professional environment came back by reaching the many somatic functions that had absorbed them. This disturbed the patient as well as the doctors who observed the symptoms *sine materia*, which troubled them enormously in the establishment of diagnoses.

In the presence of such somatic symptoms, doctors become discouraged and offer either complementary explorations or make a diagnosis of imaginary illness by referring the patient to psychiatry or a therapist to solve the problem. For them, "it's psychosomatic", that is to say, an imaginary disorder. So they forget that there is also *soma* in psychosomatics!

I followed Sandrine for a year, from November to September, in supportive psychotherapy. In fact, supportive therapy helps to develop the role of a protective shield by weakening excitations, and allowing the patient to gradually cope with daily tensions. These disorders of a "hypochondriac" nature may be without somatic foundation and as a psychosomatic therapist, our role is to repair the psychic apparatus and strengthen the mental defences to cope with the daily stress. But in some cases, these sensorimotor disorders are announcing serious disease, sometimes with a latency of several years. We must be very careful about hypochondriacal disorders.

Sandrine came to some sessions accompanied by her husband who was waiting for her to take her home. Throughout her psychotherapy, Sandrine reported her futile visits to many doctors of different specialties whom she consulted for her disorders. I always supported her, and her mental state improved throughout the year so that at the beginning of the holidays we decided that at the end of September we would bring our therapeutic meetings to a close. I had strongly encouraged her to return to work part-time, which at the time seemed compatible with the new balance of her condition. As a therapist, in such a sensitive case, it was very difficult for me to develop a strategy of modifying the narcissistic mental defences which pushed the patient to adopt an intellectual attitude in order to seek the origin of her disorders in the body. All I did was to supported her efforts, protecting her from narcissistic injuries, and trying to steer her in a resumption of her professional activities. My strategy was more of an economic and energy nature, namely redirecting energy towards the activity of work. Sandrine ended up returning to work part-time.

I have always corresponded with different doctors, insisting that the somatic state needs regular monitoring, adding that it would be important for control procedures to be implemented in order to follow the symptomatic evolution in attempting to establish or restore functional homeostasis. In my relationship with her general practitioner, I made the point in a letter:

> Dear Dr
>
> A year ago I met three times (about three hours of interview) Sandrine who had been referred to me by my colleague in the nephrology department. I will not go back over the whole file, which you know; my current diagnosis is a hypochondriac state following trauma. This trauma was not caused by the illness as such, but by the doctor–patient relationship that reactivated a trauma that has remained unconscious to this day. It is a profound narcissistic injury that results in a continuous search for the origin of somatic disorders. It is not an imaginary disorder, but a psychic reality that is not controlled by the dysfunctional mental apparatus. When the mental apparatus suffers from sharp irregularities, it cannot handle the *quantum* of mental excitations. The emotional mental excitations released by the limbic system are discharged at the level of the organs which become for all our colleagues the lines of research for a diagnosis not yet established.
>
> As a result of such trauma, my clinical experience drives me to be very careful because my hypothesis is that a hypochondriac state is a transient state occupying the time in the gap

between the trauma and either the restoration of homeostasis or the appearance of a serious illness. The lag time can, in my experience, be nine months to three years.

What to do in the meantime? We should relieve the pain of the organs by appropriate techniques that we know of or by the prescription of drugs.

I could not answer the fundamental question: what is the role played by the disease in the psychosomatic balance of the patient? It's too early, and we do not have enough anamnestic information to do this. A patient I received at the hospital had seen, during the last three years, doctors who were tired of such nomadism; I carefully examined the patient and proceeded to the psychosomatic investigation. Three functions seemed to me to be somatically problematic, and I referred him to three colleagues at the hospital. The head professor of gastroenterology has discovered colorectal cancer. The trauma of the patient went back five years. I have taken him into therapy.

I cannot tell you anything other than be patient and wait, by relieving local pain.

With the expression of my cordial, and fraternal, feelings.

Joseph: the enigma of epilepsy and his painful life

Joseph is forty-eight years old and I meet him in my psychosomatic consultancy. He is a patient who is eager to communicate and talk, while being very reserved. He immediately informs me of his concern about the discovery of thyroid nodules, which disturbs him enormously. He is very emotional and can control himself only with difficulty.

He says that he is going through a very difficult time right now and that his children are his single source of joy. He currently has them at home for the holidays. Joseph divorced two years ago and cannot get used to the situation; he has not mourned the separation. He remains very attached to his ex-wife and often thinks of her. He is not yet available for another relationship. He thinks that women are too demanding and expect an ideal man, which he does not recognise in himself. He sees this separation as a wound, a narcissistic attack. I wonder, of course, what the nature of the relationship was with his wife? What role does it play? The narcissistic wound of divorce must have reactivated another wound, which gradually appears in the anamnesis. Aged ten, he had an accident, a head trauma. As a result of this accident, he was diagnosed with epileptic seizures, and he has been taking effective medication for thirty-eight years, but he continues to have two seizures a day, accompanied by unconsciousness.

The trainee student who accompanies me in my consultation also asks a lot of questions. After consulting the patient's file, he declares:

> Doctors have not found an organic foundation to his epilepsy, which is strange, to say the least. Investigations with more modern means are desirable in order to confirm or refute the diagnosis and to review the drug treatment. In any case, he claims to be slowed down by the treatment.
>
> In addition, the announcement of the disease was very traumatic for him (it is impossible for him to do certain work, to play sports) and he rebelled against this form of "castration". It was only during his marriage that he gradually accepted this limitation. This narcissistic flaw feeds the feeling of low value and less personal accomplishment.

I am very happy with the observation of my student. It is up to me now to develop a little more the theoretical approach of epilepsy by psychoanalysis and, first, to review the medical approach that has been taken, then to make the psychosomatic synthesis of Joseph's case.

Epilepsy (Fatorusso & Rittter, 2006) is characterised by a sudden increase in electrical activity in the brain, causing temporary disruption of communication between neurons. Usually, they are short-lived. These abnormal nerve impulses can be measured during an electroencephalogram (EEG); epileptic seizsures are not always accompanied by convulsions. They are then manifested by sensations: olfactory or auditory hallucinations, with or without loss of consciousness. An epileptic seizure can occur in many circumstances: head trauma (Joseph's case), meningitis, stroke, drug overdose, withdrawal from a drug or, as in the case of my patient following the trauma, an overflow of the excitations that remain fixed at the level of the central nervous system without the possibility of discharges at the level of the somatic functions. That is my psychosomatic hypothesis.

In about 60 per cent of cases, doctors are not able to determine the exact cause of seizures: this is called essential epilepsy. It is assumed that about 10 per cent to 15 per cent of all cases will have a hereditary component since epilepsy seems more prevalent in some families. Researchers have linked certain types of epilepsy to the malfunction of several genes. For most patients, genes are only part of the cause of epilepsy. Some genes can make a person more sensitive to environmental conditions that trigger seizures. On rare occasions, epilepsy may be due to a brain tumour, a sequel to a stroke or other brain trauma. Indeed, a scar can form in the cerebral cortex, for example, and modify the activity of neurons. It should be noted that several years can elapse between the accident and the appearance of epilepsy. And remember that for epilepsy, seizures must occur repeatedly and not once. Stroke is the leading cause of epilepsy in adults over thirty-five.

Freud and epilepsy

Freud planned to write an analysis of Dostoevsky's *The Brothers Karamazov*, illustrating the epileptic writer's creativity in the early days of his life; he took a long time to do this, and in 1923 an article by Iolan Neufeld appeared, which Freud described as excellent. Neufeld put forward the hypothesis that the life and work of Dostoevsky, his acts and emotions, his destiny and his work, everything, was the culmination of his Oedipus complex. In *The Brothers Karamazov*, the father is presented as a debauchee, vain and violent; he has three sons, Dmitri, Ivan, and Alyosha. He is murdered by his fourth son, Smerdiakov, who is a bastard son who serves as a servant.

All the analysis concentrates, in truth, on the personal history of Dostoevsky and his oedipal conflict with his father, who was murdered by three moujiks. Added to this is the fact that Dostoevsky himself participated in a plot against the Tsar, considered the father of the Russian nation. All these arguments are used by Freud to justify the oedipal conflict of Dostoevsky: we have the personal history of the writer and the novel. What may have been the influence of the death of the father on the epilepsy of the writer? This is the question that Marie-Thérèse

Neyraut-Sutterman (2011) also poses in her thesis defended at Nanterre University in 1989.[9] In truth, the symptoms of epilepsy had already appeared in the writer's childhood following a major punishment inflicted by the father. Freud describes the first manifestations: they came in the form of sudden and unjustified neurasthenia when he was still a little boy. "The impression was that I was going to die immediately," said Dostoevsky later to his friend Solovieff. This anxiety attack was followed by a state that resembled real death. The first major crisis occurred at the age of eighteen when he learned of his father's tragic death.

Following the conspiracy against the Tsar, the writer and all his comrades were sentenced to prison in Siberia. It seems that this stay considerably weakened, if not eliminated, the symptoms of epilepsy that were gradually replaced, during his second marriage, by asthma. Freud had always been very ambiguous about Dostoevsky. He declared that in the face of the problem of the creative artist, psychoanalysis must, unfortunately, surrender. In a letter to Reik, Freud says:

> You are right ... in suspecting that, in spite of all my admiration for Dostoevsky's intensity and pre-eminence, I do not really like him. That is because my patience with pathological natures is exhausted in analysis. In art and life, I am intolerant of them.
>
> (Freud's letter to Reik, 1929, Freud, 1928d, p. 196)

Freud carefully studies the personality of the writer and he carefully reads the opinions of some of his contemporaries in this respect where the confusion between the creator and his creatures takes place and concludes: "It comes from his choice of material, which singles out from all others, murderous and egoistic characters, thus pointing to the existence of similar tendencies within himself" (Freud, 1928d, p. 178). See also Bonaparte, 1958; Schmidil, 1965; and Freud's letter to Stefan Zweig, 19 October 1920 (1961, p. 339).

Freud compares Dostoevsky to the barbarians of the great migrations who killed and then did penance, in an image where one catches glimpses of a mythology of the Mongol and the Russian soul. We will

---

[9] I attended this thesis defence to which my colleague M.-T. Neyruat-Sutterman invited me.

leave behind Sigmund Freud's moral opinions vis-à-vis Dostoevsky because our interest is in the importance of epileptic symptoms in the writer. Let us examine what Freud has to say about Dostoyevsky's epilepsy: Dostoyevsky's epilepsy represents neurosis, not because it is a neurosis like hysteria, but because it was a "hystero-epilepsy, that is to say, a severe neurosis". Freud raises the question of the authenticity of the writer's crises; he then suggests that epilepsy is pre-existing and that "the epileptic reaction" can be at the service of neurosis and the epileptic seizure then becomes a symptom of hysteria that transforms and adapts it!

Freud respects biological and physiological medical data. There are two epilepsies: one, organic, where the psychic life is subjected to a disturbance caused by an external cause—giving birth to real epileptic crises; the other, emotional, which makes the patient a neuropath whose disorder is the expression of the psychic life itself, hence the false seizures of Dostoevsky; in these cases it would be hysteria. He describes in this respect epilepsy on the same model as hysteria.

> It is as though a mechanism for abnormal instinctual discharge had been laid down organically, which could be made use of in quite different circumstances—both in the case of disturbances of cerebral activity due to severe histolytic or toxic affections, and also in the case of inadequate control over the mental economy and at times when the activity of the energy operating in the mind reaches crisis-pitch. Behind this dichotomy we have a glimpse of the identity of the underlying mechanism of instinctual discharge. Nor can that mechanism stand remote from the sexual processes, which are fundamentally of toxic origin: the earliest physicians described coition as a minor epilepsy, and thus recognized in the sexual act a mitigation and adaptation of the epileptic method of discharging stimuli.
>
> (Freud, 1928d, pp. 180–181)

Sigmund Freud's explanation raises many questions: he addresses the problem of epilepsy without ever referring to the excitations that assail the central nervous system by causing a major neuronal discharge. Dostoyevsky's oedipal conflict seems doubtful to me because there is no reference to Dostoevsky's genital psychosexual development nor to his desire for his father's wife! There is nothing about the mother's desire or father's wish to evict. The analytical material to which he refers reflects the violence of a boy's reactions to a brutal father who traumatised him. One can understand then that many literary critics have deeply doubted this oedipal conflict. To kill the father but not to replace him, that is what can disturb the classic oedipal psychoanalysis. In this case, it is about killing the father who is an aggressor. Can there be another explanation? First in psychoanalysis, then in integrative psychosomatics.

The hypothesis of Sándor Ferenczi

As for psychoanalysis and especially the origins of integrative psychosomatic, I will first refer to Sándor Ferenczi. In 1921, Sándor Ferenczi challenged the exclusively psychological explanation of the mechanisms of epilepsy. He thinks of it as a regression to a very archaic level of organisation accompanied by a total discharge of internal excitations by the motor pathway. This is a regression to the intrauterine situation as described by Grunberger (2003). The epileptic patient goes through a range of regressions from the situation of infantile omnipotence to the intrauterine situation. In Ferenczi's opinion, the illusion of the womb goes even so far that an epileptic in crisis is very sensitive to respiratory function (asthmatic symptom). The illusion of the matrix needs, in order to maintain itself, a minimum supply of oxygen coming from outside. If we block this intake, the epileptic is forced to wake up and breathe through the mouth, just like the new-born at birth must change environment: from the passage of the intrauterine economy to the external economy where the respiratory function starts.

For Ferenczi, epilepsy occupies an intermediate place between transference neuroses and narcissistic neuroses. He also shows that the theory of epileptic regression makes it possible to understand the relationships between epileptic seizures and the state of sleep. Moreover, referring to the nostalgia for absolute rest, evoked by states of epileptic seizures, he suggests that this may be a more or less serious attempt at suicide by suffocation! It is interesting here to recall the breathing difficulties which, towards the end of Dostoevsky's life, seemed to replace epileptic disorders.

The explanation of integrative psychosomatics

In integrative psychosomatics, the first hypothesis is that of a high quantum of excitement that goes beyond the psychic apparatus, and we must search for its origin. Joseph was the victim of a traumatic accident causing epileptic seizures and loss of consciousness. Excitations due to head trauma remain fixed at the level of the central nervous system (CNS), overloading it excessively. The function of the CNS is to facilitate the neuronal discharge causing the epileptic seizure; we can see in a great many cases that the CNS tries to use as complementary outlets the sensory and motor functions that will absorb the excitations. One can thus understand the losses of knowledge that will facilitate a return to the equilibrium of the CNS. These are natural physiological reactions of the CNS. I will add that for Joseph his divorce probably refers to maternal rejection in the early stages of life. We are in the presence of the original trauma: an unwanted child. His fear of women comes from her first maternal rejection. How in these historical conditions, which cause fixations in the process of psychosexual maturation, can a psychic apparatus develop?

It was the same with Dostoevsky who, at a very young age, suffered the violent aggression of the father which can then, in Melanie Klein's sense, be considered a "bad object". Dostoyevsky's imagination was able to develop brilliantly, but not the oedipal conflict. My hypothesis is that for him the father is an aggressor that must be killed. He may have had an oedipal element in his participation in the plot against Tsar Nicholas I. So much for the explanation of the second enigma that I present.

Nicolas: a strange amputation, return from the past

I participated for a long time in the diabetology staff where I presented, as did the doctors, the report of my visits to the patients in the service. Degradation of the health of diabetic patients sometimes leads to difficult decisions to be made to treat and save the patient.

The Professor, head of the department, had asked me to examine Nicolas because we had to make a serious decision.

I met Nicolas several times, and colleagues were waiting for my review to rule on amputation and its consequences. The patient refused this amputation that was necessary for his survival. He had neuropathy, retinopathy, and nephropathy with severe heart problems: the prognosis was poor. I found the patient in a state of drowsiness that was difficult to overcome; he went back to sleep every time I spoke. I decided to proceed with our interview when the effects of the "Stilnox" had worn off and I counted on the doctors to organise this. I was able to talk to him later. He was seventy years old: he thought he was living his last moments and had reached the end of his life. But what had been his life? Why did he think he was going to die?

Nicolas had had an interesting life until his retirement. He had been a sailor on a large luxury liner, and his eyes sparkled when he told me that he had gone around the world four times, more than 50,000 miles each time. He thought his life had been exciting and he should have written a book. He had seen many things and his human experience was great. He looked at me and said, "I can die now." He was out of breath talking to me and I did not always understand what he was saying. Nicolas is married; he has a son with whom he had quarrelled; he is happy now because since he has been hospitalised, his son has come to see him; a kind of reconciliation, but I do not know what was behind the dispute between the two men. In the background, I perceive the emotions of Nicolas, who seems confused; this disturbs him a lot. Nicolas has a great capacity to associate past and present events, thus revealing a good psychic functioning. But then, why diabetes?

Suddenly, because the therapeutic relationship is opening up an associative path and lifting buried memories, Nicolas tells me about his childhood: during the war, in Paris in July 1942, Jews were arrested and locked up in the Vél d'Hiv (the Vélodrome d'Hiver). His parents, uncles, aunts, cousins, and cousins were driven away to disappear forever at Auschwitz: he was then almost twelve years old. He grew up ignorant of Judaism and turned his back on the violent past that had taken his family away. Nicolas is inhabited by this traumatic past; I will never know how he survived by hiding his Jewish identity that now resurfaces in the therapeutic session. We understand better that he relives the current situation in the light of the loss (amputation) of his parents: the phase of mourning resurging on the occasion of the loss of a part of the body. How to prepare him for this loss and the psychic modification of the image of the body? Psychic pain is occurring not as a result of the bodily pain, masked by the drugs, but in the mental recovery induced by the interviews.

The work of the mourning of the parents and the mourning of his bodily integrity, and the return to a terrible past enlightening the current decision, ended up lifting many psychological obstacles: Nicolas, as a result of our therapeutic work, made the decision have the amputation, and I was able to inform my fellow doctors, to whom I reported the painful events of Nicolas' past.

The surgeon was able to proceed with the operation. Psychic pain or moral suffering is not here in the continuity of bodily pain but is necessary to prepare for the process of mourning.

Recall here the studies of Kübler-Ross (1969) on the confrontation with death of a sample of four hundred subjects in a state of terminal illness:

- The first phase of shock and denial;
- The second phase of anger and resentment towards those around you (those who represent health);
- A third round of bargaining to save time;
- A depressive phase;
- A last phase marked by acceptance.

These stages are fundamental so that the psychic apparatus can gradually create favourable conditions for adaptation to a new situation. My hypothesis is that these five stages take more or less time according to the degree of mentalization of the subjects. Some will remain in Stage 1 or 2 and suffer from a major depression,[10] and will enter progressive states of disorganisation without involvement of the psyche: the body alone and its defence mechanisms will be solicited, the pain is purely bodily reactivation of situations of distress from the first stages of life, with diffuse anxieties and somatic behavioural reactions. Stages 3, 4, and 5 are more related to the mourning process and its development. I do not think these steps are covered by all individuals.

---

[10] An example of "depression without an object"—Dr Pierre Marty's concept.

The stage after the amputation is also to be considered because it is accompanied by manifestations of aggressiveness whose range is broad and deserves thorough study. Nicolas goes through a stage in which he strongly criticises the medical profession and the nursing staff: he feels like "a hollow radish tossed about by waves", he resists the latent post-operative depression by a passive attitude that worries the doctors, who have again returned to me. What should be done? Nicolas, for the moment, does not want to be fitted out with a prosthetic.

In truth, the doctors do not give him the time for a state-related recovery, which must vary according to the subject since the duration is a function of individual experience. Nicolas thinks his leg is a leek; Nicolas is now using vegetable metaphors and a pictorial language. He is ready to die, and nothing can reach him anymore. I think he wants to be cremated and, like Jean Gabin, he asks that his ashes be dispersed at sea where he spent most of his life, which has given him psychic balance for a large part of his life. He does not feel he has the energy to walk again, but the nurses put him in a wheelchair, and he feels revived. He strongly criticises the skills of the doctors who gave him his bleeding fistula. I think it makes him feel better to criticise them: it is the beginning of a control over the environment—the impulse to take a grip begins to show itself again. How to explain to physicians and caregivers, who are tired of aggressive before, that they should wait? I often explain to them that aggression is on the side of life when it manifests itself. Because the danger is that the reversal of aggressive impulses onto oneself can worsen the condition of our patients; we are then in the presence of what is called self-destruction.

Maxime: the hypochondriac disorders of a young filmmaker

Maxime is a twenty-three-year-old man who, when he enters my consulting office at the hospital, seems very agitated. He sits in his chair, and I notice that his left hand is shaking heavily. He tries to control his hands by concealing them; the flow of his speech is very fast. And after the interview and at the time of writing these lines, I feel that he has tried to seduce me by exaggerating the value of his profession, namely cinema. Everyone is fascinated by cinema!

He claims to be a film producer, works in television and claims that, at first, he wanted to study medicine. He has a huge medical vocabulary to describe the long list of his somatic symptoms. Where does this vocabulary come from? The confusion is such in the first minutes of the interview that I wonder, to myself, what he wants and why he came to see me. His parents are both carers, and they recommended that he make an appointment with Dr Stora, a psychosomatist. I end up telling myself that Dr Stora lives in Nice and that his name is Jean-Charles. Maxime must have gone online because he had a lot of information about me, while reciting my curriculum vitae! The fact that, in my first profession, I was a professor at the School of Higher Commercial Studies of Paris (HEC) seems to impress him because he himself went to a private television school of which he is a graduate. He has a very long school career and many meetings with doctors and psychiatrists! Why?

Regarding the school career, it seems that he is a very intelligent boy but not keen to follow a school curriculum, do his homework on time, or comply with the discipline of educational institutions. He graduated because he is very intelligent, not because he complied with the programme. He says that you only needed to know two or three things to pass the exam. From the age of eight, he had seen psychotherapists and, since that age, no fewer than ten psychiatrists! He has had a lot of therapy with Lacanians, who he seems to despise because, in his eyes, they are incompetent. He is currently being followed in brief psychotherapy by a behavioural therapist who is very expensive, and who seems to obtain some results in terms of the reduction of his symptoms.

Later in the session, and for ethical reasons, I tell him that I will not be able to take him into psychotherapy if he already has a psychotherapist. He tells me that it is only four or five sessions of EMDR (rapid eye movement desensitisation). It all started, he said, last April when he was on a major trip to the United States for his job, a journey in which, because he was ill, he lost all his money. It all started with vomiting, gastric discomfort, which ended him up in the emergency department, where a lot of tests were performed: scans, MRI, etc. All this without any results. The symptoms persisted and disrupted his trip so much that he had to return to France. He had no heart problems or neurological disorders; the troubles have ceased and resumed, but for the moment we cannot attribute to any event the cause of such violent somatic reactions, except the strong emotion connected with the trip to the United States. These are functional disorders whose medical origin is indeterminate for the moment.

I ask him questions about possible trauma at his birth, and he tells me that his delivery was difficult for his mother and that he was born with the use of forceps. It is a first traumatism of which I cannot evaluate the resonance in its current functioning. He talks very little about his parents, his professional environment, his relationships with others. He tells me, however, and this is a sign of an early transferential relationship, that he knows that I have written many books and that he wonders if he should read these books before engaging in therapy with me. When he was attending classes at his TV school, the teachers did not want students to watch the films they themselves had produced. I reply that his curiosity must be analysed and understood. He must try to understand what he unconsciously seeks in reading a book or a film: what exactly is he looking for? Does he need this knowledge to reassure himself? All these questions challenge him, and we end the interview so that I can assess his demand.

I see Maxime several times and, during one session, he wonders a lot about the excitement that comes over him, his hyperactivity, and all the somatic disorders that disturb him deeply. Yesterday evening, he was in bed with his girlfriend and suddenly he had an impulse to look for his teddy, his transitional object[11] because he felt he needed it; he needed reassurance. I confirm the role played by this object which protects one from excitations in the absence of the maternal object. He tells me about his mother who is visiting Paris from the provinces, and he recalls that after the meeting last Tuesday, he found his mother at home in his apartment and that he felt very uncomfortable with her, which prevented him from taking notes about the session. He also remembers

---

[11] Object chosen by the very young child that allows him to survive in the absence of the mother and to calm him; it ensures the transition before the internalisation of the maternal object that will allow him to live with the absence.

that his temperature rises during the day, often going up to 38 degrees for about 20 minutes, and then falls back down to a normal level.

All his thoughts are centred on what he evokes of his past, namely very close proximity to his mother and what he calls his repression of sexual impulses. He also mentions the fact that in pre-adolescence his father beat him.

I offer a first interpretation: the fear of coming closer to his mother has reactivated his desire to be loved by her and to love her, but such a rapprochement could be punished by the father who beats him. He accepts this interpretation, which goes in the direction of an approach to the oedipal conflict. This problem gradually begins to enter the psychotherapeutic scene: Maxime has been followed by many psychiatrists and psychotherapists! He now expresses a lot of emotion about his childhood and the tragedy of his life. As a child, he was surrounded by the admiration of everyone in his family, by his school; his teacher publicly told him that he looked great on the school photograph, surrounded as he was by thirty children. He seduced the entire school by performing in a comedy show. At the age of eleven, his parents moved to another neighbourhood and he lost the environment in which he had lived; in losing this frame he lost the admiration and the esteem of everyone who had been contained in it. That's where the drama resided.

I then offer another interpretation about his desperate search recently for the admiration of people with whom he comes into contact. I would add that this desperate search for admiration, as in his childhood, and affection (hence of maternal love), is not negative because it has allowed him to succeed and continue to be successful in life. He then recognised that being lost in this search for admiration needed considerable expenditure of energy! He continued the meeting by talking about his symptom of diarrhoea, which had ceased after last Tuesday's session; it is a symptom that temporarily resumes and disappears. I stress that the excitations that move about at the level of one's body express deep distress. He thinks that the body is for him a surface onto which he can project his anxieties. This is a very relevant observation because it is about psychic anxieties and not somatic ones.

He ends the session by telling me a dream in two parts: in the first part of the dream, he is in a peep show and he wants to make love with a woman who refuses him, then he finds himself on the floor in the company of homosexuals who discuss sex between them for a long time but, he says, "it does not interest him, it's not his thing". In this dream, we then see him in his hometown where he meets a girl from his past who has always refused him and he finds himself in a sordid place, then in a toilet; he then realises that the toilet roll has fallen into the toilet. Despite his disgust, he recovers, and urine flows slowly from this toilet roll.

The interpretations of the first part, thanks to his associations, made it possible to understand that this woman, whom he does not know and who is the object of his desire, still refers to his mother. For the first time, the issue of his relationship appears, and he understands that the prohibition of incest, due to repression, and of heterosexuality in general, direct him towards homosexual relations which he does not approve of. The second part of the dream seems more sordid. It is relative to his adolescence, to his amorous failures, and to the fact that the sex act itself is dirty; I add that the word "dirty" is not appropriate in this context and that it will be up to him to understand this dream a little better.

At the end of the session, following my interpretation, he comes back to a dream he told me about last Tuesday: his father is on all fours in front of him, his backside exposed, and he makes love to him. It's a dream that scares him. I tell him that he told me this dream the previous Tuesday, which he cannot remember. I conclude by telling him that this dream is the equivalent of his rapprochement with his father, not in a passive mode, but in an active mode; that, in any case, we will come back to all this in the work we do together. I know from clinical experience how frightening the psychic homosexual dimension can be in the analysis of what is called, in psychoanalysis, the negative Oedipus complex. We must take time.

During a session, Maxime suddenly evokes a problem that has been the main theme of his difficulties since we meet. I remember that he came to consult me at the Pitié-Salpêtrière Hospital because he had confused me with a doctor who lived in Nice and who bears the same name as me. Maxime's issue is a question of identity, it is my hypothesis: he tells me that during the holidays, he went through a very deep crisis and that he has now renounced to use the surname R. because he now wants to assume his own identity. Maxime no longer wants to use the name of a Jew to go into media and film circles; he wants to be himself. I remember that Maxime is not Jewish. But it all started in adolescence, and then especially when he left his family and came to Paris to follow the teachings of an elite film school and get into the circles that would allow him to achieve a professional career. I told him on that occasion that recently, looking at my schedule, I had difficulty putting a name in front of his first name. This simple sentence suddenly made him switch to his distant past: he tells me that he only took on his father's name at the age of eight. In his family book and his birth certificate, it is the name of his mother that first appears; it was later, at the age of eight that his father returned home, and he took on the father's name.

Part of the session is about his passive relationship with the father; I want to talk about passive psychic homosexuality, the negative Oedipus, and about the various homosexual relations where it tries, with much difficulty and pain, and against his own will, to penetrate himself anally. We work on his relationships, his fantasies about his father, and his oedipal conflict, on the passive dimension. As in many cases, some patients act things out, because the fantasies of oedipal penetration by the father seem scary.

We also come back in the session to everything that has happened to him since his trip to the United States, which was a complete failure because he got sick and, since that time, has begun to suffer, in hypochondriac fashion, various disorders including gastrointestinal disorders. Maxime interrupted our psychosomatic and psychoanalytic work to visit his family. He dies in a serious road traffic accident; he was not driving the car himself. It caused me deep emotional shock.

The case of Maxime illustrates the issue of the "name of the father" on its negative side (psychic homosexuality) with a narcissistic dimension and a somatic hypochondriac dimension that disturbed the medical diagnosis: what was suffering Maxime from?

Lucas: an asthmatic Ulysses—why so many trips?

Lucas is a great traveller; he was referred to me by my colleague Céline, president of an association. We started to meet though the year; Lucas is also a psychotherapist trained in an association with whom I have been in a teaching relationship. He is a medium-sized man, born in Belgium; he always wears a soft hat, a backpack, loose clothing, a jacket with dozens of pockets, always ready to go.

He started life on the roads of France and Belgium at the age of three months when the Germans invaded Belgium and the panicked population fled. The family eventually returned to his home village and Lucas has a moving memory of his relationship with his grandmother. He always talks to me using a notebook that he carefully pulls from his bag and in which he has written all the events he wants to talk to me about. In some way, he talks to me through his writing, but I do not understand the reason right away. It is obvious that this is how he puts me at a distance and bypasses the rule of free association. One's thoughts can only be accessed by repeating one's written thoughts and not one's verbal thoughts. This is defensive and for months I have not been able to associate freely with his writing. The psychic door of free associations and the memory of the past were somehow closed.

He is a very nice man who smiles, eager to do well and to please me. I must say that I did not always understand what was happening in the transference relationship because it made me unable to understand the unconscious dimensions of our relationship. Lucas travelled across France and Belgium for group seminars that allowed him to earn a living. At the end of his trips, he returned to Paris to meet up with me. I was curious about these trips, but it is only recently that I have understood the profound for his geographical mobility. Lucas divides his life between Anne, who lives in the South of France, and Myriam who lives in Brussels; he divorced a long time ago and met Anne ten years ago, whose life he shares when he does not travel. He has three grown-up children, one boy, and two girls. A few years ago, he and his son travelled to India to visit a monastery. He is very attracted by the spiritual dimension, which has made him travel thousands of kilometres around the world.

All the therapeutic interviews take place in the same way: he opens his notebook, tells me about Anne, her attraction to her (Anne is also a therapist) and his inability to live with her, when life could be so pleasant. It is hard to understand why after being with her for some time, he moves away, as if it is dangerous for him. He did the same with Myriam, who he left to go to South America, where he stayed a few years, always giving group lessons, which seems to me to be a mysterious activity. He sometimes reminds me of Ulysses and his Mediterranean journey. Why move so far away for so long? What about Lucas? Because it's a real character that keeps me at bay and my entire problem will be to interpret why he keeps me at a distance; why does he have so much difficulty getting closer mentally to me? What are the reasons? But does he really keep me at bay and is not the problem of a different nature? I wonder a lot about the conflicts with his two women, but I cannot understand the deep reasons, although he often talks about the two of them. Myriam is the mother of her children; she is a very rigid Catholic and a very devoted woman. But why leave her? As for Anne, she gives structure to his life and helps in many aspects of his professional life, in a small town in the South of France. She has a beautiful house where she welcomes him and he can, on the ground floor, receive patients. He sometimes goes to Spain to give courses.

In Paris, one of his colleagues puts him up in her apartment and he has a room where he can also receive patients, which allows him to follow the teaching courses, still something mysterious to me, that he must continue for many more years. What is the role played by this teaching in his peregrinations? He talks about it a lot and focuses heavily on courses that will allow him to gain more knowledge and more experience in his discipline. But here again, with his colleague, he repeats the same behaviour of rapprochement and remoteness; all these behaviours that are repeated over time end up hurting the women who welcome him, with whom he has relationships. They do not understand, and it is true that it is difficult to understand. Lucas does not want to fall out with any of them; he wants to be welcomed, accepted, and does not wish any conflict that could call him into question. As soon as he perceives a sign of discontent that does not correspond to what he expects of the person, then he takes up his bags and goes to get the train. I often think that where he feels best is on the move. He tells me dreams where he is always travelling, by car, by train, or by plane; it is either in an airport or en route to an airport or train station. Lucas travels between several centres, in at least four big cities where he has ties and where he feels good, always with the justification of either the teaching he gives or the follow-up of patients in psychotherapy.

At the last session, Lucas arrives as usual but does not pull out his notebook. He sits lowering his eyes and does not look at me for the whole session, which is strange in view of his behaviour in previous sessions. He tells me that he has made some serious decisions: to move from Paris to the town where Anne lives and settle down with her. But after he had packed all his belongings and left the Paris apartment, causing great upset to his colleague, he could not leave, as if afraid to live with Anne. In this latest meeting with Anne, he had stressed her repressive and intrusive aspects, which does not correspond in any way to her vision of the world and relationships with others. Suddenly, Anne had become different from the image he usually had of her. Such a discovery made him stay in Paris; but after doing what he did, Lucas regrets the gesture and wants to get closer to Anne. At the same time, he had met up with Myriam and offered to live with her. After making such a proposal, Lucas, frightened, asserted the opposite to Myriam who felt terribly hurt by his attitude. Within a week, three women resented him so much that he was rejected by all of them. Lucas had wanted to reconcile himself with each of them and the result was contrary to his expectations.

During this session, I first thought of a masochistic dimension: Lucas did everything to make the other become an aggressor and reject him; in this way he had their love and a pathological masochistic pleasure, since they rejected him. But he did not follow such a line and put himself elsewhere; the associations concerning his travels in the past brought him back first to his mother's wanderings in Belgium and then to being sent away from his family to cure his asthma in Switzerland, in a boarding school. Then comes the remembrance of all his movement and the removal from his parents from early childhood until adolescence.

I then gradually realised that if the maternal object was introjected, the so-called distance from the object had not been internalised because of early trauma. When a conflict arose, unable to take a mental distance from the other, Lucas moved geographically, as Pierre Marty (2006) taught us in his remarkable contribution to the allergic object relation. This is the mystery of this "Ulysses", forced into countless geographical displacements to escape unresolved conflicts. Just like the baby he was, he kept moving on the roads.

Marc: noise and silence—how to explain the headache of the patient?

Marc was referred to me by a colleague and long-time friend; she met Marc in a big brasserie in Paris while she was sitting at table with a friend. He complained of long-standing migraines and headaches, and she recommended that he meet with a psychosomatist.

I met him several times during the first month of therapy: he is a very tall man; he is bulky and strong. Marc is a very intelligent man who grew up in a family where they worked a lot. His mother, born in 1936, is a rigorous, very demanding woman, who instilled in him an ideal life to which he continues to conform. Marc is between forty-five and fifty years old: I will specify his exact age later. On the side of his mother, it is a family of intellectuals since the father of his mother was a university professor who was politically engaged. As for his paternal grandfather, to support his family he worked all his life in two professions: one, during the night, was that of hospital porter; the other was during the day. He himself belonged to a large family since he had nine sisters. His father was suffering from a serious illness, and I never discovered what had become of him. Marc did not talk about him further.

Marc has suffered from migraines since resuming work in September following the summer holidays. I try to reconstruct with him the story of his life, to understand his symptoms. He is a very attentive man: he associates well and tries to understand what is happening to him. I gradually put words to the symptoms he is suffering, while justifying my remarks and declaring to him that, for the moment, these are hypotheses to allow us to better understand his behaviour, especially the absence of thought in his head which is blocked, annihilated, by the migraine symptoms.

Marc works in a big brasserie and he manages everything for a boss, who is also a friend. He works nearly fourteen hours a day without a break and suffers from major insomnia. I begin to link the migraines of early September to the resumption of his work and the question of whether he had really wanted to go back. I must add that during the month of September, the migraines were very violent and lasted all day. During October and November, Marc was gradually forced slow down at work and then to take time off; he came to see me in early January. I stress the turning point between the holidays where he was able to rest and the resumption of an activity that he loves so much, but which so absorbed his energy that his body could no longer keep up.

He agrees on this point, and he is now considering in his sessions the need to end his current work activity and to take up one that suits him better. There is the potential conflict with his friend who is the boss who runs the brewery; his difficulty in expressing his disagreement, saying no, has resurfaced. I immediately think of the inhibition of the aggressive drives underlying somatic symptoms at this stage of the integration of the "no", described by René A. Spitz (1965).[12]

Marc cannot cope with conflict. He tells me that he is always the first to "calm the game". Once calm is restored, he can face things, and speak, but he avoids conflict at all costs, and the same goes for the management of staff at his place of work. It has been like this all his life in the context of his family; Marc has two older brothers and in our last session we talked at length about his past because he has no memories before the age of sixteen. Nothing about childhood, nothing about adolescence!

Today's session was particularly illustrative because progressively we come to identify some components of his problem. Marc arrives very relaxed; since this morning, he has not had a migraine. He intends to leave next Monday for two weeks holiday in Asia and I congratulate him, wishing him a happy holiday. In fact, since our last session, he has suffered from migraines for only two days a week. He had taken refuge in the castle of one of his friends, who did not require that they ate or spent time together, which allowed him to relax completely. For the first time, he tells me, he has barely answered the phone and has lived

---

[12] Spitz establishes the presence of three stages of development of the object relationship in children: the pre-objectal stage of the first three months of life, characterised according to him by the non-differentiation between the baby and his mother; the stage of the precursor of the object, marked by the appearance of the smile (third to eighth month); the stage of the libidinal object (eighth to fifteenth month), when the child differentiates his mother favourably from other people. From the fifteenth month, according to Spitz, the child goes into nonverbal communication and begins to use the "no", which marks the birth of the autonomous self.

in silence. What he wants, by the way, is silence and tranquillity, and it is what he will find on a distant island in Asia where he has rented a villa.

The fact that he insists on silence makes me think of noise; at that moment, our interview takes a different turn, since he comes back to the sound of his childhood and the noise of his workplace. About his childhood, he tells me that his mother had told him that his migraines had appeared when he was nine years old. Marc had lived in a small apartment, and he shared a room with his two other brothers, the eldest of whom made a lot of noise and listened to hard rock all day long. How can you live in silence when, in one room there is music blaring out, and in another his parents are watching the television at full volume? The only place he could go was the bathroom, where he read throughout most of his childhood and adolescence but has no memories of that period.

I then advance the hypothesis that migraines have appeared to protect him from noise; in this way, he cannot hear anything because at that point there is so much going on in his head. I also stress his relationship with the noise, which he wishes would go away but from which he does not want to be separated. He confirms my interpretation because, throughout his professional life, he has worked in very noisy places: nightclubs, brasseries, etc. He lived in noise, while hating it. Unconsciously, he has always searched out noisy places, in a repetition compulsion that continues today. He agrees with this suggestion, and he reflects on his future. Leaving the current brasserie would be a difficult step because his boss is very attached to him and his dedication to the job. Marc managed to get his boss to accept his departure and is currently working on the accounts and looking for a successor. Marc is a fighter, a very active man. I told him that in my opinion, his body sounded the alarm at the beginning of September because it was saturated, in a state of nervous exhaustion. He understands this hypothesis and confirms it. I tell him that his body has not been spared and that, therefore, the only way he can continue his life is to start thinking again about how to protect himself rather than having migraines. I add that he should thank his body for protecting him. Migraines are also a defence system.

I try to extend this hypothesis to various periods of his life and our next sessions are devoted to this exploration and reconstruction of his past, to restart the psychic system.

We return to his ego ideal and his emotional life: he tells me about his son and the fact that he was very rigorous with him and that he helps in his studies. Marc is divorced and his son lives with his former wife. He has good relations with his wife, and we can understand this, since Marc does not want any conflict. He disagrees about his son's current life with the daughter of one of his friends who is a rather lax mother; this has affected this girl who often meets up with Marc and relates to him as a kind of father substitute.

After his relationship with his former wife, Marc had met a woman who shared his life and left him a few years ago. This woman was a manager at the brasserie, a woman of action who certainly did not suit him and who used him since he was the general manager. It is obvious that we will have to explore the difficulties of his relationships with women. At present, Marc is following his son's studies closely; he can meet with him more often since he is not working and is now much more available to him. His son is studying in a University Technical Institute (IUT) and he is taking parts of his exams; his results seem excellent. Marc encourages his son to carry on.

At the end of the session, Marc informs me that he feels good, that he has no migraine symptoms, and that he feels liberated. I wish him a happy holiday.

CHAPTER 5

About the originality of psychosomatic psychotherapies

Can the mind[13] heal the body? How does the psychosomatic therapist treat the mind in a complementary way to the doctor who heals the body?

In the first four chapters of this book, I have presented fifteen cases proposing to demonstrate the complexity of the interrelationships between psychic functioning, neuronal functioning, and somatic functioning. This is a methodological approach that will be explored in this last chapter, addressed to patients and, especially to therapists and physicians, who wish to take this path.

The power of the mind has profoundly influenced many therapeutic movements since the beginning of humanity. Even today, traditional therapies, which are in the majority globally, develop techniques and rituals in which the spirit dominates. It is the same in the psychoanalytical approach to somatic patients, developed in the different schools of psychosomatism in the twentieth century. The capabilities of the psychic system and its different modalities of functioning strongly

---

[13] The mind has two dimensions: a rational and cognitive dimension, and a psychic dimension.

influence the therapeutic process. The somatic, real body is primary and, in the long run, benefits from the benign functioning of the mind in its psychic component.

During the different stages of psychosexual development, somatic functions and organs are progressively invested with the libido or psychic energy, and psychoanalysts and psychosomatists speak, at that moment, of the "psyche-ised" body; it is obvious that all the investment failures by libidinal energy of the somatic body will weaken the overall functioning. We now better understand the predominantly psychic orientation of therapies initiated by psychosomatic psychoanalysts.

This fascination with the domination of the mind over the body led my first steps in psychosomatics. Then, after creating a psychosomatic consultation at the Pitié-Salpêtrière Hospital, I understood, through my years of practice, that the problem was much more complex. I first proposed the following paradigm: "The human being is a psychosomatic unit." The mind or psychic system participates, alongside the central nervous system and various somatic functions, in somatic disorders. There is not, therefore, according to this hypothesis of psychosomatic illness, any suggestion of "imaginary" psychical causes for diseases; conversely, any disturbance of somatic homeostasis disturbs the psychic functioning. One cannot separate one from the other: the mind-psyche and the body. If we accept this global approach, then we understand that all diseases are psychosomatic and that the body and mind, each according to their own modalities, participate in somatic, and therefore psychosomatic, disorders.

In our societies, the body, in allopathic medicine, is treated by doctors, and the mind by therapists. At present, there is no teaching in the faculties of medicine about psychic functioning; there are tentative advances in the relationship with the patient, body-relaxation techniques, and, in some cases, mindfulness meditation. As for the mind, in the faculties of psychology and clinical psychopathology there is no teaching about the relationship between the mind and the body. In 2004, my psychosomatic teaching in the University of Paris 8 disappeared; it was replaced by the teaching of the University Diploma (DU) in the Faculty of Medicine of Pitié-Salpêtrière, which terminated in 2015.

In integrative psychosomatics, the "psychosomatic therapist" has as his main concern the repair of the psychic system so that it can again metabolise and "work through"[14] the external and internal excitations assaulting the psychosomatic unit. The aim of therapeutic work is, first, to dampen the psychic excitations that daily assail the psychosomatic unit of the patient. Gradually, the psychosomatist will help the patient to establish, or restore, links throughout the psychic system that have been affected by the traumas of life events: undoing the links between mental representation, affects (emotions and feelings), and behaviours.

The work of the psychosomatist can only be accomplished by considering somatopsychic organisations. I proposed to complete in my work on neuro-psychoanalysis, the stages of the psychosexual development of the Freudian model by indicating very clearly that these stages are carried out within the framework of the integration of the central nervous system coordinating somatic functions. So, I have developed a new model that I describe as "neuro-psychosomatic", extending to the central nervous system and somatic functions and organs. The scientific advances of the late twentieth century and the beginning of the twenty-first century in neuroscience and medicine have allowed me to propose a new meta-psychosomatic model. The psychosomatic therapist treats the psyche in its relation to the central nervous system and somatic functions. We are no longer in the psychic system in the strict sense.[15]

This adjustment has been illustrated by all the cases presented in this book because it consists of linking mental representations, behaviours, and affects (emotion, and the feeling of an emotion). As for the "somatic" doctor, he is responsible for treating the patient by prescribing drugs or using surgery. In integrative psychosomatics, these two caregivers must work together to repair the psychosomatic human unit. The "therapist" doctor of the mind-psyche must work "hand in hand" with the somatic doctor; to better guide the direction of psychosomatic treatment, medical data should not be ignored.

---

[14] "Psychic elaboration" (*Durcharbeiten* or "working through") refers to the work of the psychic apparatus to control the external and internal excitations that assail it daily. To do this, the therapist aims to interweave mental representations, emotions, and behaviours; it facilitates the abreaction or discharge of emotions.

[15] As in the model of Pierre Marty and other schools of psychoanalysis.

A brief return to the history of the body and the mind

The division of the body and the mind was proposed by Anaxagoras in the fourth century BC with the clinical and theoretical consequences of there being either the body (allopathic medicine) or the mind (Sigmund Freud and metapsychology). It was not until nearly twenty-four centuries later that we finally had a model of the functioning of the mind, thanks to Freud. But the path leading to a model uniting body and mind continued with the approach of psychosomatic medicine (Franz Alexander) and the inspiration of the psychosomatic psychoanalytic (Pierre Marty). Each of these two approaches is based on the predominance of one discipline over the other: the predominance of medicine or the predominance of psychoanalysis in the explanation of somatic disorders or somatisations. The question arises of how medicine can explain what is happening in the mind, whereas this discipline has never developed a knowledge of how the mind works! Or to know how psychoanalysis in the strict sense can explain somatisations, whereas the real body has never been developed in the model of metapsychology. In both cases, we are confronted with the epistemological limits of the disciplines.

I will indicate later the theory that I propose to connect medicine, psychoanalysis, and neuroscience. I developed this theory at the end of the twentieth century and particularly in the first ten years of the twenty-first century. As far as psychoanalysis is concerned, it is important to point out immediately that the Freudian genital stage (the oedipal conflict) is very rarely addressed in psychosomatic therapies. My clinical hospital experience with more than 4,500 patients suffering from various pathologies revealed to me a psychic functioning of a pregenital nature and very often of an archaic nature (in early life), illustrated by the cases presented in this book. We were in the presence of adults, and we had first to treat in them the child who had not grown up. None of my masters in psychosomatic had taught me. The maternal figure in all its dimensions was the key to the psychic functioning of somatic patients.

I then turned to the many contributions of Melanie Klein, Donald Winnicott, René Árpád Spitz, W. R. Bion, and Daniel Stern, who became the teachers of what I called integrative psychosomatism. It will be understood that a new metapsychological model must be built, taking into account the archaic and pregenital dimensions of the development process of psychosexual maturity.

Psychosomatic therapy

In January 2014, I offered my colleagues at the Integrative Psychosomatic Society a training seminar on psychosomatic psychotherapy. I recall that in June 1993, following the death of Pierre Marty, founder of the Institute of Psychosomatics, of which I was chair from 1989 to July 1992, I created, in the university hospital group of Pitié-Salpêtrière, a psychosomatic consultancy, localised in endocrinology, symbolically attached to the psychiatric service,[16] and welcoming patients from all departments of this hospital. This consultation ended in January 2015 and allowed me to develop a new approach to psychosomatic integrating the three disciplines: medicine, metapsychology of archaic and pregenital phases, and neuroscience. No one thought more than twenty years ago of a scientific theory that could interconnect disciplines.

Treating the body without healing the mind is an incomplete process, which can help us understand why so many people continue to be sick after their apparent healing! We are faced with a very serious question as to what the role played by disease in the psychosomatic balance is. How do we explain why many patients consider that they have not been properly treated or that they are not cured of their disease? How do we encourage chronic patients (more than 20 million of them in France) to observe medical prescriptions? Often, these patients give up taking their medication, to the dismay of allopathic doctors. What can be done? These questions draw our attention to body disorders in relation to the mind. We can also ask what has occurred at the level of the psychic system,[17] which is, I have repeated several times, a defence

---

[16] I would like to thank Dr Alain Braconnier, who put me in touch with Professor Jean-François Allilaire, head of the psychiatric department, who helped me considerably in my first administrative steps.

[17] I recall that the psychic system is constituted during the first twenty years of life by the interrelation between mental representations (of things and words), emotions, and behaviours. This system is, like the immune system, a defence system; it is also interrelated with the central nervous system (Stora, 2011, on neuropsychoanalysis).

system analogous to the immune system. Why has the patient not been able to stop the daily excitations that assail him and which, ultimately, are at the origin of the somatisations?

Personal history: the need to know one's unconscious

I began to practice classical psychoanalytic treatment from 1973 as part of my training in the Psychoanalytic Society of Paris, after long personal psychoanalysis. I continued this training until I qualified. My vocation to treat somatic patients was reactivated by my psychoanalytic practice and, on the advice of friends, I met Pierre Marty at the Institute of Psychosomatics (IPSO). For five years I trained in this institute with Pierre Marty who taught me how to treat somatic patients. I was able to undertake with him, starting from his "method", the first epidemiological studies;[18] I have pursued these to this day by completely renewing the model that I call "meta-psychosomatic". This type of training leaves a very strong impression and I have, in one of my books, talked about the "psychoanalytic Superego" developed by the training members of the Paris Psychoanalytical Society so as to adopt standard psychoanalytic behaviour. First, in my opening remarks, I want to pay tribute to my late master and friend Pierre Marty who died in June 1993 at the Pitié-Salpêtrière Hospital, which became for me a symbolic place, the place of realisation of his wishes—to develop psychoanalytically inspired psychosomatics in the hospital—and the birthplace of integrative psychosomatics.

When I first arrived at this hospital, I began by clinically examining patients from the IPSO training but, over time, my observations have evolved profoundly and, aware of the shortcomings of this training, I understood that I needed a much more scientific method to explain somatisations. As I no longer had contact with Pierre Marty, my clinical and theoretical point of view gradually evolved to discover a theory of somatisations that his psychoanalytic model did not explain. I must admit that the School of Paris has proposed important psychosomatic concepts that continue to be the basis of some of our reflections in integrative

---

[18] See No. 3 of the *Journal of Psychosomatics* devoted entirely to studies and epidemiological research in psychosomatic, thanks to the model that I developed.

psychosomatics: essential depression, operative thought, ideal self, progressive disorganisation, behaviour neurosis, allergic object relation.

The somatic unconscious and the repressed unconscious

Unlike in classical psychoanalysis, the psychosomatist is confronted with two human unconsciouses: the organic or somatic unconscious and the repressed unconscious. When the psychic apparatus is overwhelmed by external and internal excitations, these are transmitted by the central nervous system to reach the somatic organs (according to our new theoretical approach). Two types of somatic disorder must be distinguished. The first is the one that Freud developed in 1893:

> The symptoms which we have been able to trace back to precipitating factors of this sort include neuralgias and anaesthesias of various kinds, many of which had persisted for years, contractures and paralyses, hysterical attacks and epileptoid convulsions, which every observer regarded as true epilepsy, *petit mal* and disorders in the nature of *tic*, chronic vomiting and anorexia, carried to the pitch of rejection of all nourishment, various forms of disturbance of vision, constantly recurrent visual hallucinations, etc.
>
> (Freud, 1893h, p. 4)

On the model of hysteria, Freud shows us very clearly that the irreconcilable representation is made harmless by transposition (conversion) of the sum of excitations which is linked to it in the body (Freud, 1895b). It is important here to differentiate conversion hysteria and psychosomatic disorders: patients with psychosomatic disorders are very different from those with psychic disorders. This was commented on by Michel Fain at the psychosomatic symposium of All Saints' Day 1967 and raises the question of psychosomatic disorders according to psychopathology and that of the difference in the structural organisation of patients suffering from either somatic disorders or psychic disorders in the strict sense of the term.

Psychosomatic questioning seems to be limited, on the side of the psychic universe, by Freud's concern to create a metapsychology, emerging from a psycho-physiological point of view, and, on the side of psychosomatic theorists and practitioners, by the relations to be established between erotic bodies and sick bodies, between sexual urges and instincts of conservation, with the aim of creating concepts that allow somatic patients to be approached. Now we cannot approach somatic patients without clarifying the epistemological problem of the place of conversion hysteria in psychosomatic thought; in other words, should the psychosomatist take care of patients suffering from conversion hysteria? There are diagnostic difficulties: our clinical practice reveals that it takes a psychoanalyst, a psychiatrist, a clinical psychologist, or *a fortiori* a doctor, a very long time to differentiate between hysterical and psychosomatic disorders; our observation, in this respect, elides with the experience of many psychosomatists. What about psychic excitement in conversion hysteria? In Draft E of 6 June 1894, Freud (1894) describes, regarding questions about the birth of anxiety, two distinct phenomena of innervation:

> In hysteria, it is *psychic* excitement that takes a wrong path exclusively into the somatic field, whereas here it is a physical tension, which cannot enter the psychic field and therefore remains on the physical path. The two are very often combined.
>
> (Freud, 1894)

From this quotation, we can summarise the theoretical hypotheses by provisionally concluding that: (1) there is a physiological, non-sexual dynamism; (2) that psychosexual development, from fixation points, confers erogenous zone value on an organ or a function; (3) that the somatic alteration caused by the disease of an organ or function may eventually confer the value of an erogenous zone, thus offering support for the symbolic expression of fantasy, but also contributing to the maintenance of repression. At this point, thanks to the alarm signal activated by the organic anxiety, we have a mechanism that allows doctors and therapists to question organic disorders and for the psychosomatic therapist to start a work of connection between body and mind. It is important to put words on things, that is, to connect sensory perceptions and their verbal meanings, so that the psychic system can gradually restore the protective function, as far as possible, of the body.

We must understand that in anxiety neurosis the excitation is at the level of the body (functions and organs) and that it cannot be discharged psychically while remaining in the bodily domain. There is no elaboration.

All organs and functions of the body have sensors that regularly inform the central nervous system of any changes occurring. This eventually results in what is called an anguish alarm signal that is very difficult to understand because it is expressed by symptoms that only doctors can decode, as far as is possible. When the body speaks, it is very difficult for a human to understand what it is saying! I will end by still referring to Freud regarding the attitude of the psychoanalyst therapist and doctor:

> To put it in a formula: [the analyst] must turn his own unconscious like a receptive organ towards the transmitting unconscious of the patient. He must adjust himself to the patient as a telephone receiver is adjusted to the transmitting microphone. Just as the receiver converts back into soundwaves the electric oscillations in the telephone line which were set up by sound waves, so the doctor's unconscious is able, from the derivatives of the unconscious which are communicated to him, to reconstruct that unconscious, which has determined the patient's free associations.
>
> (1912e, pp. 115–116)

I will add that medical data are fundamental to complete the reading of the repressed unconscious. The combination of medical data and psychic functioning data will make it possible to establish a diagnosis and a direction for the cure.

What in my approach has changed with respect to Pierre Marty's theory? I gradually noticed that the Paris School did not take into consideration the somatic functioning of patients; once diagnosed as a failure of the functioning of the psychic apparatus, somatisation took over, as if everything depended on the proper functioning of a psychic apparatus fully formed at the end of the psychosexual maturation process! The Paris School did not take into consideration the medical dimension of the patient, the real body of the patient. Now, we treat the somatic patients first with the real body and not the "psyche body", that is, the body psychologically invested by the libido. The first training of psychosomatic psychoanalysts was the "classic psychoanalytic cure"; this model has strongly influenced the thinking of these early psychosomatists who were then thinking in terms of planning the classic treatment for somatic patients.

Psychosomatic psychotherapy was thought to originate from the classical cure. This classic cure was developed by Freud for "classic" neurotic patients; it was, therefore, patients fixed in an oedipal genital position. Observations of patients and somatic patients revealed that these patients, as part of the psychosexual maturation process, were fixed in archaic problematic positions of relationship to the mother in the first months of life and/or in pregenital positions (oral and anal). These deficiencies in the process of psychosexual maturation led to the conclusion that the psychic system was not fully constituted and that it did not have the capacity to handle the quantum of daily excitations that assail us.

Moreover, in some cases, transference neurosis had not developed in the first six years of life. We are in the presence of fragile human beings that we can describe, as André Green (2009) suggests, as non-neurotics, a description recently adopted by psychosomatists and psychoanalysts in their writing. It was therefore not a question of adapting the classic psychoanalytic treatment, but of developing appropriate therapeutic techniques for these patients. We can no longer speak of a transfer in imitation of classical psychoanalysis, but of attachment to the meaning given by Bowlby.[19] All these findings led us to develop new techniques and new therapeutic strategies.

The indications and contraindications of psychosomatic psychotherapy concern the somatic patients dominated by their behaviour, with great poverty of their imagination leading to associative difficulties

---

[19] British psychoanalyst who developed the theory of attachment that inspired us strongly in the psychosomatic approach to the archaic phase of development. He exposed his theory after the work of Winnicott, Harlow, and Lorenz (ethnology). He explored the relationship between a young child and his mother; the child needs to develop, he says, a relationship of attachment with at least one person who takes care of him in a consistent and continuous way to experience normal social and emotional development. This relationship precedes the internalisation phase of the object.

necessary to the therapeutic treatment. We are once again in another model of psychic functioning of human beings.

For patients with great poverty of the imagination and dominated by their behaviours,[20] it is not possible to treat them in psychosomatic therapy, because the associative capacities are often non-existent, and thus render the therapeutic work impossible. This is a contraindication; we recommend that psycho-corporal psychotherapy be started from which it will be possible, after a year or two, to treat them face-to-face by developing their associative psychic abilities. For some other patients, who are not in the "current and factual" account of the events of their lives, it is possible to take them into therapy, which will be conducted by a psychosomatist who will lend, as Bion says (1961), along with Pierre Marty, his "thinking apparatus" to think thoughts.

The face-to-face technique

In contrast to psychoanalysis, the somatic patient faces the psychosomatist therapist (a face-to-face relationship rather than a couch–chair relationship). Somatic patients are very fragile and cannot lie down and risk aggravating their symptoms. Face-to-face is highly recommended in the relationship to a therapist who adopts a warm and empathic maternal attitude. It is important to be very careful in the relationship and in future interpretations; the therapist manages the quantum of excitations during sessions and builds psychic abilities to allow patients to mentally resist the trials of everyday life. It is a question of providing continuous support for life instincts to increase the capacities of resistance.

The medical dimension is fundamental: the knowledge of the diseases of our patients from childhood to the time of their examination must be taken into consideration and analysed very carefully. If you are in a hospital, it is better to consult the patients' medical file only after the psychosomatic investigation and, I prefer to add, after the first elaboration of the case. If you are not in a hospital, contact the general practitioner, and, if they refuse to give you information, it is best to contact the patient to have sight of the information in his possession.

---

[20] See a brief note in Appendix 3 on behavioural neurosis.

You must inform the patient that this will greatly assist in the process of the therapy. This way of working allows psychosomatic psychotherapists to better understand the patient's experience of the illness by relating the history of illnesses to the history of life events. The patient will also feel that his real body is also taken into consideration by the therapist.

Is it possible to establish a psychosomatic diagnosis? The diagnosis is made by the consultant in less than two hours of investigation, which is a feat because it is to assess "the essential vitality of an individual". It goes without saying that the clinical know-how and the knowledge of the consultant are in great demand. Pierre Marty[21] developed a classification and a nosography for the diagnosis. I proposed an epidemiological study to assess the ability to establish a diagnosis from his nosography. Were psychoanalyst therapists at IPSO able to make a diagnosis based on the knowledge of their initial training? I will only repeat in this chapter some of the findings of this study and, in Appendix 2, you will find the nosography of integrative psychosomatics that I propose for establishing a diagnosis.

The results were surprising but consistent with the primary training: 94.4 per cent were of neuroses of character, 1.9 per cent of neuroses of behaviour, and 2.2 per cent of essential allergic organisations. Five sections of the nosography had been used on the ten existing ones. I put forward two hypotheses to understand why there were so many neuroses of character. Hypothesis 1: the consultants, deeply influenced by their first psychoanalytic training, mainly retained only neuroses of character. Hypothesis 2: the sample of the hospital was representative of the French population where neuroses of character predominate. To complete this information, it is important to know that 177 patients had symptoms of one somatic disease, eighty-seven of two diseases, thirty-eight of three diseases, and seventeen of four diseases. For 263 of these, 81.4 perc cent were of the lesion type, and for fifty-seven of functional type.

---

[21] For Pierre Marty's nosography, you can consult the special issue of the *Revue de psychosomatique intégrative* of May 2018 devoted to epidemiological research in integrative psychosomatics. The new integrative psychosomatic nosography is in Appendix 2. Website: www.spi-int.com

I would like to remind you that these were the first years of implementation of the "Pierre Marty" classification and that, presumably, the consultants had had difficulty in assessing the level of individual mental functioning. For what reasons? Some investigators hate the "mental void" (no association of ideas). Consequently, this may explain that after having classified eleven cases of neurosis of well-mentalized character,[22] it is possible after six months to detect eight neuroses of character with uncertain mentalization and three neuroses of ill-mentalized character. In contrast to the first investigators, other researchers seek at all costs to see mental emptiness in as many cases as possible: out of sixteen cases of neurosis of character with uncertain mentalization, eleven have been reclassified into neuroses of well-mentalized character; similarly, of four cases of behavioural neurosis, two were reclassified as well-mentalized neuroses.

The fundamental structure, which identifies the diagnosis of neurosis more or less well mentalized, was considered by Pierre Marty as incapable of being removed in adulthood, therefore constant over time. Is this still so? We will carefully examine the new integrative psychosomatic nosography in Appendix 2. What is in question here is the perception of the observer trapped by his countertransference, to which is added the multiplicity of criteria qualifying a mental functioning.

The countertransference must always be carefully analysed by the therapist and one can add unilateral or reciprocal seduction, or rejection leading to improve, or evaluate the appreciation of, neuropsychic functioning. The impotence of the investigator may unknowingly and momentarily revive the mental functioning, and blind him … All these remarks must lead us to develop the analysis of the countertransference of the psychosomatist. The descriptive criteria of the "fundamental structure" are numerous; they rest on the psychosomatic theory apprehending the two Freudian topicals[23] and the preconscious qualities.

---

[22] Classification Pierre Marty: cf. the third issue of the *Revue de psychosomatique intégrative*.

[23] A psychic process is described by its three coordinates: dynamic, topical, and economic coordinates. This is the three-dimensional point of view of psychic phenomena. The malfunction of the first topical, by deficiency, discontinuity, or disorganisation, should arouse attention in that it often preludes the appearance of somatic disorders or shows the risk of aggravation of these disorders.

In fact, during an investigation, there are more than fourteen macro variables to evaluate (see Chapter 1). The high number of criteria, the difficulties inherent in the differentiated functioning of the two topics, and the difficulties of perception of the observer, caused by the countertransference, shed light on the reality of the mental functioning of the psychosomatist: a functioning appeal to associative thinking and logico-rational functioning.

This continual back-and-forth does not facilitate mental development and may, during the clinical investigation, be at the origin of the important loss of information. Diagnostic errors are low among psychosomatists with long clinical experience: also following my research on the clinical practice of psychosomatists, I gradually developed during the ten years following the death of Pierre Marty a new classification to make the work of diagnosis and investigation of psychosomatists more comfortable (see Appendix 1 and Appendix 3). But my research work was far from finished because the explanation of the processes of somatisation rested entirely on the capacities of the good functioning of the mental apparatus. The body only participates secondarily in the case of somatisations. It lacks a discipline to be able to better understand the transmission of unprocessed excitations by the psychic apparatus to the different somatic functions, namely the neurosciences. We are, in truth, at the epistemological limits of the "psychosomatic" model developed by Pierre Marty.

The contribution of neurosciences

I started to study neuroscience in the early 1990s. Progressively the fields of the three disciplines came together in a synthesis that I was able to establish only with my publication of the book *La Neuropsychanalyse* (Stora, 2006). I was interested in neuroscience because Freud had tried, at the beginning of 1895, with "Project for a scientific psychology" (1950a), to lay down the neuroscientific bases of what was to become psychoanalysis. But he realised that the knowledge of the period he lived in was insufficient to provide him with the scientific neurological basis for what will be called "psychoanalysis", so gave up and his essay was only published after his death (in 1950).

I wondered a lot about this, then I met the North American and British colleagues of the International Neuropsychoanalysis Society who had founded the movement in New York. They brought together leading specialists in neuroscience and psychoanalysis to launch it, and it now has several thousand members in twenty countries around the world. Edelman, Damasio, and other neuroscientists were among those who founded this international association, along with Professor Mark Solms, who was its first president. I would like to point out that when the university diploma of integrative psychosomatics was created, Mark Solms agreed to be a member of its scientific committee.

The fields of psychoanalysis, medicine, and neuroscience have come together. I started to make the synthesis within a model that has been developed over the last twenty years, and which I have called "the theory of the five systems". I wanted at all costs to give a solid scientific basis to this new approach by calling upon the systems theory of Ludwig von Bertalanffy (1969).[24] These three disciplines have quite different scientific development rhythms and are very different from each other. It is difficult to establish the interrelationships, but this is possible. We can examine patients in their psychic, medical, and neuronal dimensions by associating the context of life events and somatic disorders. This is the method that was finally developed; in some cases, but not all, neuroscience is possible; we know that the hypothalamus is at work in many pathologies. It is important not to rely exclusively on psychic concepts, as far as psychosomatic psychotherapies are concerned.

I did not limit myself to Freudian metapsychology in the strict sense; in psychosomatics, we have found that the psychic problems of somatic patients are related either to maternal deficiencies at the first stages of life, or to pregenital fixations, or to failures in the first six to seven years of life. To do this, I turned to eminent psychoanalysts to establish the foundations of a metapsychological model that synthesises all their contributions. They are Melanie Klein, René Árpád Spitz,

---

[24] In 1937, Ludwig von Bertalanffy (1901–1972), a biologist, presented the concept of an "open system" that will gradually evolve towards the "General System Theory". The purpose of this general theory was to find explanatory principles of the universe considered as a system by which we could model reality. He said: "There are systems everywhere. This means that objects with the characteristics of the systems can be observed and recognised everywhere. That is totalities whose elements, in dynamic interaction, constitute sets that cannot be reduced to the sum of their parts. The psychosomatic unit is a complex system."

Donald Winnicott, Wilfred Bion, Daniel Stern, André Green, and Bernard Golse. It is this model that I use for the establishment of the anamnesis, the diagnosis, and, finally, the therapeutic course.

Psychosexual maturation process and neuronal development process: integration of both systems

Referring to the archaic phases of development I have, for example, developed in depth the structure of the core of the self, the precursor of the self. The self-nucleus consists of the following: immune, neurological, and psychic components. Freud told us that the first self was a bodily ego, and he stopped there; from the work of immunology, neurology, and eminent contributions of the aforementioned analysts, I considered it important to develop the notion of self, constituting the foundation of the ego. It is a fundamental step during which the identity of the individual and the difference between self and non-self is built.

To this theoretical and clinical element, I have added the following propositions: the process of psychosexual maturation of human beings is always accompanied by a process of neuronal integration. The integration of the two systems is necessary to complete and establish what I call "psychosomatic unity". If there is no maturation of the neurological system, the psychic system cannot develop; the psyche can only develop from the neurophysiological and biological basis. This "autobiographical" dimension (Damasio, 1999) is fundamental because it is the receptacle of the identity of an individual: who are we, where do we come from, what is the history of our family, etc.?

The self allows us to exist in time and space, to remain true to who we are. One can understand, for example, the dramatic cases of adopted children, since the components of the self are deeply related to the first days and the first months of their lives. The education of children in the context of adopted parents can provoke conflicts and divisions within the self, conflicts that will reactivate during adolescence and leave adults and parents helpless; in truth; they do not understand what is happening because it is a problem of a search for identity. It is the same for all of us because we all have stories containing problems around the constitution of our first identity. This identity core has immune and neurological components. It is important now to recall a number of recommendations, and some advice, before addressing the issues of therapeutic cure.

What diseases and which patients can be treated today by psychosomatic therapists?

The new psychosomatic approach is appropriate for patients suffering from any known pathology. The psychic system participates to some degree or other in all somatisations. There is no such thing as a psychosomatic disease in isolation; it only exists once it has reached a living being. It is important that physicians reintroduce the psychic system into the psychosomatic unit. We are not truly in the twenty-first century if we follow the way of questioning of the theorists and clinicians of the twentieth century. It is important that the psychotherapist has done some work on himself (in psychoanalysis) and that they work with an understanding of the subconscious in the relationship with the unconscious of patients. Clinical psychologists and psychoanalysts in the strict sense must resort to psychosomatic training. One cannot improvise in curing somatic patients.

A psychosomatist must first know the basic functioning of his unconscious, but also of his preconscious and finally of his ego ideal and his superego. This way of proceeding is unusual for a psychoanalyst trained in an institution because such a training focuses only on the analysis of the oedipal conflict of classical neurosis. The knowledge of preconsciousness is assumed, and the superego problem is treated in the context of oedipal triangulation. This is not the case in psychosomatics. The preconscious, the place of connection of representations of things and representations of words, is strategic in the evaluation of the psychic functioning of somatic patients; it is the place of the imaginary whose wealth and/or poverty is assessed; the poverty of the imaginary reveals that the psychic system is not going to treat (elaborate) the excitations that will flow in the four neuronal systems[25] before reaching the somatic organs and functions opening the way to somatisations.

---

[25] In neuroscience, there are four fundamental subsystems of neural control of emotions: the exploratory system, the reaction system of rage and anger following aggression, the fear reaction system, and, finally, the separation-distress system or the panic

It is important to analyse the ideals programmed into us by parents, by the social milieu, and by the culture of our country. We can have several cultures in ourselves that must have been analysed and accepted (the ethno-psychoanalytic dimension). These are future constitutive elements of the superego. When one is facing a patient, one can find oneself solicited at all levels of psychic functioning: at the level of our unconscious, of our preconscious, of our ideal of the self, and of our superego. Our imaginary is constituted in a certain environment that will structure our unconscious and preconscious; we must accept and understand the different imaginaries we face in the therapeutic process. The confrontation of the imaginary can trigger countertransference that we will analyse if we want the process of psychosomatic psycho-therapy to develop.

As for our superego, the more we have analysed and resolved the oedipal conflict, the better for our patients; I say this because during the therapeutic process we can make countertransferential judgements that will disrupt the therapeutic relationship. The first recommendation is not to pass judgement on our patients, knowing that during treatment, we can make behavioural and cognitive recommendations. I am refer-ring here to the therapies of narcissistic neuroses, addictions, and the sensorimotor dependencies created by them. We are at a very archaic level where the interventions and not the interpretations are of a behav-ioural and cognitive type. In this way, we can take the place of parents and make life recommendations to our patients. We ask patients ques-tions about how they live their lives and we need to take some impor-tant precautions here because we are on the razor's edge: patients come to us to be a little more independent, to be more able to take decisions for themselves. We have a parental role that we will have to resolve at the end of psychotherapy so that our patients can move away from us. The introduction of laughter and humour into psychosomatic therapies can play a very important role in easing the superego relationship or that of the ego ideal.

---

system related especially to the feeling of loss and sadness (see Panksepp, 1998). My hypothesis is that the quantum of excitations, depending on the nature of the object loss or aggression, is transmitted to one of the four subsystems (see Stora, 2011 for more information).

When it comes to welcoming patients, we need to know how to position ourselves in front of them and how to get in touch with them. Psychosomatic therapies take place face-to-face; sensori-motorism is required because the patient, to the extent that he or she can look at us, observes our physical appearance, our mimicry, and our emotional reactions. As we know, there is a nonverbal communication from unconscious to unconscious and what we feel will be felt (but not put words) by the patient. Projective mechanisms on the part of the patient may be manifested revealing that he can see us as a persecutor; he can make fantasies of all kinds of characters. In the therapeutic relationship, we play all roles in truth, just as in psychoanalysis, induced by the compulsion of repetition. The difference with psychoanalysis is that we are in the perceptual field of the patient, which facilitates the process of identification[26] at the centre of the relationship. Since I speak of perception, I want to evoke the first system of the Freudian model: the perception-consciousness system which will be strongly referred to. The main goal of therapy is, at the end of the process, to increase and broaden the patient's perception-consciousness system. As the therapeutic work progresses, the field of his consciousness will increase. The patient will take a different view on his life, his relationship with himself and others; his vision of the world will be profoundly changed. At this point in my presentation, it is Freud's recommendations that come to mind: what are these recommendations?

We are dealing with somatic patients, and it is their bodies that we also take care of; the medical dimension of the sick body will be added to the psychic dimension. Doctors have been trained to observe and treat patients' bodily diseases; their listening can be disturbed by their initial training since they have to switch from a medical cognitive field to looking for symptoms belonging to the listening field of psychic functioning. Only a doctor who has been analysed can operate this shift of listening within his psyche and, later, interpret the words of the unconscious. This listening will enable doctors and psychosomatic therapists

---

[26] This is a psychic process in which mirror neurons play an important role. The subject appropriates certain aspects and parental qualities, thus progressively constituting the components of his personality.

to better understand the disease and the role played by the disease in the patient's psychosomatic balance.

The other dimension to consider is the management of cancer patients and patients with serious diseases. The therapeutic management of too large a number of seriously ill patients can eventually put the psychosomatist in difficulty. Health and mental balance are threatened by the excess excitement caused by the care of these patients. The emotional overload can compromise health; the recommendation is therefore to limit the number of very serious patients in the psychosomatist's practice.

A psychosomatist must be careful in choosing patients: not to fall sick oneself is an important objective. My criticism now, considering the recommendations that I have just made, will address the approaches of psycho-oncology, psycho-neuro-immunology, etc., that is, therapeutic approaches modelled on medical disciplines, while integrative psychosomatic is transversal in nature. The psychic system has its own specificity on the epistemological level, and it cannot be the subject of specific partitions such as medicine. Its only specificities are those concerning very young children, adolescents, and adults. There is no specific psychic functioning for a somatic disorder: cancer, migraines, gastroenterology, etc. We cannot define a specialist therapist of a somatic disorder as we do in medicine. Here again, we are dealing with an epistemological problem that needs to be clarified. This is why I am opposed to any specialisation of medical discipline in the integrative psychosomatic approach. We must remember that it is a question of putting in relation a psychic apparatus, the central nervous system, and the somatic functions.

What about the somatopsychic?
The theory of the five systems

If I speak of the somatopsychic relation, it is because doctors unfamiliar with the integrative psychosomatic approach evoke this question: what about the somatopsychic? I would first like to remind you that the terms psychosomatic and somatopsychic were coined by Dr Heinrich Heinroth in Vienna in 1815 and 1818, but that these two approaches have been widely questioned, first by psychosomatists of analytical inspiration, and today by integrative psychosomaticists who developed the model of the five systems—the psychic system, the central nervous system, the autonomic nervous system, the immune system, and finally the genome—between which there are dynamic interrelationships. This approach makes it possible to understand that, whatever the imbalance of a system, it will call into question the global homeostasis, and after a certain delay, the homeostasis of the five systems can be found *without* a return to the initial condition of equilibrium. There is never a return to the origin in the physical sciences in the same way that we cannot go back to the origins of humanity except phantasmatically!

Why the theory of the five systems? It was important that the new discipline named "integrative psychosomatics" be based on an unquestionable scientific basis. In the case of my first thesis, I was acquainted with the works of Karl Ludwig von Bertalanffy,[27] who developed a general system theory in 1937; the concept of the "open system" that he proposed gradually evolved into the "general system theory" (von Bertalanffy, 1969). The purpose of this general theory was to identify principles that explain the universe as a system, with whose help we could model reality. Von Bertalanffy declared: "There are systems everywhere." It is then possible to arrive at a hitherto unsuspected unitary conception of the world. Whether one is dealing with inanimate objects, organisms, mental processes, or social groups, everywhere similar general principles emerge. Von Bertalanffy partnered with economist Boulding, physiologist Gérard, and mathematician Rapaport to found, in 1954, the Society for the Study of General Systems whose objectives are:

> to search for the isomorphism of concepts, laws, and models in the different domains, and to promote their transfer from one domain to another; to encourage the development of adequate theoretical models in areas where they are lacking; to promote the unity of science by improving communication between specialists.
>
> (Checkland, 1981, p. 93)

---

[27] Cf. note 24 on Ludwig von Bertalanffy.

There may be unexpected systemic frustrations caused by life events that reach the psychosomatic unit in a traumatic way. Psychologically, we need to examine the functioning of the patient's psychic apparatus and the therapeutic strategy that can help us restore a certain balance. Reinforcing the patient's self to restore balance does not mean in any way a "cure". Healing patients is another problem. I insist here on the main role of the psychosomatic therapist which is that of providing excitement-shields in the image of maternal behaviour.

Direction and duration of the cure

The problem that I want to develop now is that of the direction and duration of the therapy because I am often concerned about the duration of psychoanalysis and psychoanalytic therapies when I hear patients say that their therapies lasted ten years or even fifteen years! According to somatic pathologies, the duration of psychosomatic therapies is quite variable; depending on the level of psychosomatic fixation helping us to establish a diagnosis, we can establish a direction of the cure and a duration that allows us either to reinforce the fixation to restore the disturbed balance, or to go through one or more stages of the process of psychosexual maturation. I would like to point out that, from the beginning of psychosomatic psychotherapy, the process of psychosexual maturation can resume its advance, and it is the reactivation of a neuronal and genetic process. It is then up to us to take the patient from one stage of development to another stage; for example, in the context of the metabolic syndrome where there are strong oral fixations, the direction of the cure is towards the integration of the anal stage so that the patient can have better drive control of his eating behaviour. This integration takes a long time, and the question will arise from the continuation of the drive integration process: should we be directed towards the phallic and genital stage? Should we take a therapeutic break to wait for the stabilisation of the condition and the improvement of the patient's health? Therapeutic periods that are too long can strengthen the psychic and emotional dependence of the patient by weakening his capacity for autonomy.

Pierre Marty often spoke of an indefinite duration of psychosomatic psychotherapy; this refers to very fragile patients who have been stabilised, whom one can meet once a month or once every two or three months in order to support their "life events". For the other patients, we can make an assessment at the end of therapy and leave the door of our office open and keep all other means of communication (phone, email, etc.) available. It is important that psychosomatic psychotherapies be conducted in a satisfactory way, free from the censure of the psychoanalytical approach in its strictest sense. The technique of psychoanalysis, as far as we know it from being analysed ourselves, must not disrupt our functioning as a psychosomatist, but rather contribute to a better knowledge of our unconscious in relation to somatic patients; each of us must continue his self-analysis, the analysis of his dreams, the analysis of his countertransference in order to better understand the relation to the patients (for example, why we might feel aggression towards the patient).

Apart from a better knowledge of our unconscious, of our preconscious, of our superego, and of our system of values, we appeal to the different theoretical-clinical models, which constitute our only working tool; it is important, then, to move from the theoretical model to the clinic itself, to what is happening in the session. What did we hear in the patient's words? What have we heard from his unconscious? How can one place the words in the context of the course of the cure to determine the direction of the therapy? How is the patient living his illness? What is his or her relationship to the body? There are problems of the development of the psychic image[28] of the body alongside to the neuronal image of the body; the problem of identification with the patient, and especially understanding his defence system. We must understand the role played by the defence system in the overall balance, as the disease can also be a defence. Then there will be the problem of care and healing; if we have not analysed the defence, we cannot cure the disease medically without risk of symptom displacement. The doctor will tell the patient that he or she is cured while the psychic problem has not been resolved; then a new disease will declared itself!

---

[28] The psychic image of the body develops throughout the process of psychosexual maturation, the libido investing the body and opening the way to desire and pleasure.

The economic dimension

The patient's economic dimension must always be kept in mind in order to better understand their ability to invest in their life and their environment. The economic dimension has two components: a somatic energy component derived from metabolism, and a libidinal component, which is the psychic energy invested in the relationship to others and/or in different activities. When a human being is sick, the disease absorbs some of the energy that is concentrated in the organ or function in difficulty. It is quite possible that the depression of the patient is due to a large decrease in the quantity of energy at his or her disposal. In addition, it is essential to evaluate the resources and investment capacities of psychic energy in different activities in order to better assess vitality. These are indications of the economic dimension that will allow us to better treat patients.

Is it possible to reconstitute neural circuits in the context of a psychosomatic therapy? During my clinical experience with patients in neurology departments, I worked a lot with Emma, whose case I described in Chapter 2; she was a brain-damaged patient and my job consisted in reconstructing neural networks damaged by her glioma. The neuroscience approach allowed me to conduct the demonstrated psychoneuronal therapy. Emma did not have access to her working memory, preventing her from remembering the tasks she had performed professionally (she was a librarian and could no longer write out the reading sheets for her books). How to build new circuits in memory was the challenge I faced in this therapy, and I relied heavily on the concept of brain plasticity to reactivate new neural networks. There is nothing magical in such work; therapy requires between nine and eighteen months to develop new neural encodings. I used the motor activity cortexes to access memory networks related to hand movements. By writing the reading sheets for the books, Emma was able to memorise, and use, her specific circuits to help the readers of the library.

To understand the patient, knowledge of neuroscience is fundamental, as is medical knowledge of diseases. It is important to establish an initial psychosomatic diagnosis, to complete it with a medical diagnosis, preferably by making contact with the doctor of the patient, and to retain what the patient says of his illness, to know what mental representation her or she has developed. You must also get the patient's consent if you want to contact their doctor. I was recently referred to a patient with cardiac myopathy; I was worried about such a diagnosis, which I had come across when I did research on cardiac transplants in the Pitié-Salpêtrière cardiology department. The assessment of somatic risk is fundamental for a psychosomatist, hence the need to contact the cardiologist of such a patient once permission has been obtained. This ties in with my remarks about psychosomatic risk and about the difference with the psychoanalyst because we do not have the same risks. We live with the risk of seeing our patients die, which is a very tough challenge for a psychosomatist therapist.

I had taken into treatment a patient suffering from very significant asthma attacks that had several times precipitated a coma; I first received him in my office, then, as a precaution, I decided to follow him in the hospital setting, which provided more security in case of a crisis. It is up to us to evaluate for each patient the psychosomatic risk in all its dimensions. We must work safely for the good of our patients. It is up to us to know what the diseases and pathologies of our patients, and the risks related to these diseases, are, and if you are not a doctor you must obtain as much information as possible.

The number of sessions, missed sessions, holidays, and payment

Psychosomatists do not function like doctors, nor do they work like psychoanalysts. For the number of sessions, first evaluate psychic functioning using the psychosomatic risk assessment method (see Appendix 1), then after taking the patient's history, establish a first diagnosis that you can review after six months of the course of therapy. The anamnesis can take place over one or two sessions, which allows you to take stock, then propose a rhythm (once a week, once every fortnight or once a month). You must be very didactic with the patients, that is, explain to them what the therapeutic process is, and what you expect from them in the work of the relationship. It is best to talk to patients empathically and warmly, to gradually teach them how to work as a patient. It is important to address the behavioural dimensions, their lived events, and associate them with their emotions. I remember a film that was set in the desert in Arizona. A car stopped in front of a cafe planted in the middle of the desert. The character entered the cafe and was brought a menu.

On the menu, strangely, is written, "Why are you here? Are you satisfied with your life? Are you afraid of death?"

Is it not, after all, these questions our patients ask themselves when they come to meet us? In the unconscious background of their visit, there is first, for the somatic patients, a medical approach: "Repair me, doctor." In a way, our patients indicate the direction of the cure: repair the psychosomatic unit, find a sufficient and satisfactory balance of energy. The main objective that we pursue is at the level of the drives of self-preservation, the level of medical and psychosomatic repair.

We must always have in mind the goal of developing "insight"—that is, the patient's lucidity about the relationship to his body, his illness, and how to live his life. It is, as I said earlier, to broaden the perception-consciousness system of the patient. What does the patient perceive in us? What is he projecting unconsciously onto us? What role do we play in his attachment or transferential relationship? What does he see on our face and in our behaviour that reminds him of unconscious behaviour? It is important to pay close attention to the rhythms of the speech, the silences, and the shifts from present to past tense: invite the patient to talk about the events of his current life, then take a current event and associate it with emotion and behaviour in order to fully relive the scene described by the patient.[29] Then try to reactivate, as far as possible, the past of a few years ago and, gradually, go back in time. It is a long and difficult job; some highly invested words can open the door of the past and reactivate it. We can, without our knowledge, take a path dictated either by our countertransference or by the projections of our patient. We must have analysed ourselves clearly enough to understand what is going on and to accompany the patient in a new way.

To question oneself is fundamental for the therapeutic process; we must question our perceptions, our assumptions; we must constantly question ourselves. We must also be sufficiently lucid and flexible to question our first hypotheses. Very often, the somatic patient goes initially to the medical part, to review all the somatic disorders of his life. We must be very patient in listening to disorders that may have never been heard by doctors. We must also be attentive to the emotion

---

[29] This is the process of association of ideas.

accompanying the story of the troubles revealing the suffering. This is a defence system that uses medicine to avoid talking about oneself.

The problem of the therapeutic process is going to come up since it will be necessary to move from somatic symptoms to the associative capacities of the patient; how to restart the psychic system is a fundamental question. The somatic disorder can hide a defence since the somatic symptom will open the door to relationships maintained by the patient with his parents and his environment.

About the defence system

Throughout the therapeutic process, we must constantly pay attention to the patient's defence system. This is our main work combined with multiple interventions and interpretations that will challenge the defence system and expand the perception-consciousness system. I am thinking about a patient, in therapy for three years, now fixed in an archaic traumatic position due to a maternal deficiency in the first year of life. In psychosomatic therapy, we often have cases of maternal deprivation; if the transfer neurosis[30] cannot be developed in the first six years, and the maternal image is not internalised, it is the attachment relationship that will prevail in the first years of therapy. It is obvious that the therapist—male or female—will have to be very comfortable with their feminine dimension (psychic homosexuality). One cannot become, during the therapy, the mother of a patient if this dimension has not been deeply analysed. This is a problem of identification and of the regression of the psychosomatic therapist. My patient, in the early days, attacked me endlessly, and this aggression was sometimes accompanied by projective forms, since she saw disturbing-looking heads on both sides of my

---

[30] The absence of the oedipal organisation means the shortcomings of the constitution of the infantile neurosis with fixations at the different stages of the pregenital organisation. One cannot speak of infantile neurosis before five to six years in reference to the oedipal phallic stage. For Sigmund Freud, regarding "Little Hans": "I am therefore tempted to claim for this neurosis of childhood the significance of being a type and a model, and to suppose that the multiplicity of the phenomena of repression exhibited by neuroses and the abundance of their pathogenic material do not prevent their being derived from a very limited number of processes concerned with identical ideational complexes" (Freud, 1909b, p. 147).

own head. These hallucinatory forms reflected the level of deep regression in my patient; an expression of its psychotic core without being a manifestation of psychosis.

She made me play the role of an aggressor, and what she expected from me as the sessions and the development of her associative capacities progressed, was, through the reconstruction of her personal history, that I reject her violently, just as her mother had, not only during the first year of life but also in the years that followed. I was forced into playing the role of persecutor and, momentarily, I accepted this role to better understand the defence system based on the patient's primary masochistic core. The patient could only receive love and affection from a human being who was persecuting her. The development of an object relationship allows the defence to be interpreted. The problem was more complex in the case of this patient because of addiction involving sensorimotor fixation in the early stages of life, sensorimotor fixation by which libidinal haemorrhage was manifested daily, since the psychic apparatus was not closed at one of its extremities. The patient could not live alone with herself, drugs keeping her company morning and night.

I succeeded, over years and by the construction of the story of her life, in linking all the elements that then allowed me to progressively establish milestones leading to the interpretation of what is known as the "reversal of sadism on one's own person". This is the first form of expression of masochism related to maternal rejection; the psychiatric approach of talking about alcoholism is very simplistic when one assumes that an addiction is replacing the maternal object. My hypotheses refer to the traumatic relationship of an aggressive mother replaced by a self-destructive addiction. It is the person herself who turns his aggressive impulses against herself as if to give "life to her life".

A psychosomatist therapist must be able to withstand, for a very long time, thanks to the mechanisms of his masochistic core, the aggressions of the patients until the opportune moment of the interpretation or interpretations which will dismantle the whole system of defence to draw out a stronger self. It is work that is often exhausting, but quite exciting. You are constantly challenged in your abilities to move between past and present, in your capacities for regression, and in your ability to communicate rapidly with your own subconscious. We must be able to explore our psychotic core and come back brutally to the genital level by going through the whole process. We do not always understand what is happening, and we often need two to three months to understand the unconscious psychic processes. How do we live in the meantime? How do we maintain the therapeutic movement? How do we bring up new material? This is a complex, multi-level job. Imagine facing a self-destructive patient: what would be your reaction? Your countertransference is strongly in-demand because it is a terrible emotional situation and difficult to bear. Imagine yourself, then, in the role of an empathetic and warm mother who sees her child destroying itself because this is the therapeutic situation that the patient is going to demand of you.

A psychoanalyst is in a relatively comfortable situation sitting behind the couch in silence; but a psychosomatist is strongly solicited and he must, in relation to the psychoanalytic technique in the strict sense, modify his device and often switch to what the Americans have developed, namely the intersubjective interpretation (Boston Change Process Study Group, 2002; 2004; Bowlby, 1969; Damasio, 1999). This is the interpretative system that I adopted some twenty years ago; the patient triggers in us a sudden emotion that it is up to us to understand since it refers to events in our own life generated by this same emotion. These events echo the current problem of the patient of which we are the mirror; the patient cannot relate to what he is feeling, but if we are aware of the events of our own lives, we can, by carefully choosing how to illustrate the feelings, help the patient to understand them. Awareness of the intersubjective relationship will allow links to be established and facilitate the resurgence of associative chains related to the most distant past. A new dynamic will emerge, thanks to intersubjective interpretations. Intersubjectivity will fill the void of the preconscious since in this way we will lend our "thinking apparatus" (Bion, 1961). We will fill up, with our own life, that of the patient. Is this not, after all, what a mother does with her child in the first years of life?

We, psychosomatists, represent benevolent parental images, and we will often accept from our patients certain actions which have never been accepted by the parents. I say all this with great care because in our patients there is always a child that we must protect from destruction. But the fact that we are different will allow the self of the patient to grow and become stronger.

My patient's projections onto me are often meant to turn me into an odious or aggressive person, which allows her to continue living inside her system without questioning it. We must be able to assume the roles of being sadistic, being bad, and we must accept all roles until gradually they open the eyes of our patients. How long can we withstand such an ordeal? It all depends on our psychic resistance, our patience, and especially the narcissistic identification with the patient. Only an interpretation, at the appropriate moment, makes it possible to undermine the resistance and the defence system; it goes without saying that throughout a psychosomatic therapy we make very few interpretations, but when we do they are intended to establish links between the associative chains that have gradually emerged from the preconscious.

We have an important job to do, namely, to restore the links of the psychic system between mental representations, affects (emotions and feelings), and behaviours. It is a question of constructing, by the reactivation of memories, the web of a psychic life which had been reduced to the utterance of facts devoid of imaginary. Thanks to progressive remembering from earliest childhood to the present, we are able to identify the character of the persecutor that has become incarnated in the different beings she has encountered during her development and professional life. Once the entire preconscious framework has been reconstructed, it is possible to state a series of interpretations on the "in the same way as … then likewise …" mode that will make it possible to undo the pathological links established over nearly forty years. It is an analytical interpretation, very structured. The patient will demonstrate reactions that Freud described very well, namely that the patient will reject our interpretations, and that he will be in denial; a defence system of an intellectual nature may appear. Patients will do everything to deny and destroy our interpretations. The important thing, in this case, is to be convinced of our interpretations, to resist, and to put up with questioning our intellectual capacities. It is a question here of constantly analysing the countertransference following the interpretations. Here, we are back in psychoanalysis's favourite place.

It is obvious that you must be convinced of what you do, how you do it, and when you do it. If we make a mistake, we recognise it very quickly and try to correct it. If the interpretation is relevant, do you still rely on Freud's experience of resisting the criticisms of the patients until they accept the relevance of our work at all levels of the psyche? It will be the beginning of a psychic mutation.

James Strachey (1934) is the author of an important research work on mutative interpretations. He described a privileged interpretative mode whose purpose is to encourage, in the context of the therapeutic process, the demonstration of instinctual impulses, particularly aggressive impulses, thus leading to a profound change in the neurotic organisation of the patient. The psychosomatic therapist, because of the therapeutic relationship (attachment), is the object of the unconscious projections of the patient. If all goes well, the patient becomes aware of the gap between the aggressive nature of his feelings and the therapist's attitude; the patient will gradually recognise that there is a difference between the original fantasy object and the actual external object. The patient, realising that the external object does not have the aggression which he attributes to it, reduces his own aggression towards the object, allowing him to introject a less aggressive object. As a result, his archaic superego will become less aggressive, and the patient will have increased access to the material of his infancy. It is important to note that Strachey emphasises that it is essential that the analyst's attitude remains based on the analysis of the countertransference and that it does not become a direct emotion expressed in reality. For him, the continuing risk of the therapeutic situation is that it is transformed into a real situation. The therapist then becomes, unknowingly, a real object and the patient can no longer project onto him his fantasies of seduction or aggression; the therapist will lose all ability to interpret and cause the necessary changes to help his patient.

The fight against resistances, the defence system, can be challenging, especially when you are in the presence of the patient as infant. We often despair, and sometimes we can question ourselves about our professional practice. How long will it take for patients to go through this long psychosexual path from childhood to adolescence and reach adult genital age? We must here call on the neurosciences to understand that the subjective interrelations with the patient, the creation of this space consisting of two people, and between two people, gradually reactivate the process of psychosexual maturation in close relationship with psychosomatic organisations that I hypothesise in my book on neuro-psychoanalysis (Stora, 2011), that is to say, that we reactivate the neural circuits related to the maturation of the different erogenous zones of the body. The process goes through regressions at the various attachment points and, once the most archaic point is reached, we can resume the forward movement and control the process.

The number of sessions

The establishment of a first diagnosis in the psychic and somatic dimensions allows one initially to propose the number of sessions necessary for an effective psychotherapeutic to be followed. The pace of the sessions is important to maintain the movements of the unconscious and to support the energy of our patients: a session or two a week, a session every two weeks, one session per month. In truth, we can only work in psychosomatic psychotherapy at the rate of one session a week, at least for the first and second years of therapy. The main objective is the resumption of the psychic functioning and the improvement of the patient's vital strength.

The price of the session

The price of the session is set based on the average market price and what you expect for your professional income. The price of the session also depends on the patient's income and what he is willing to pay you. The advice is to take on only 10 per cent of your total patients at a reduced rate; this is the same ratio as for high-risk patients.

In France, psychiatrists and general practitioners practicing psychosomatics can arrange reimbursements if they have agreements with social security organisations. Some GPs and psychiatrists have a practice of charging the price of sessions with a refundable portion and a non-refundable portion.

Duration of sessions and missed sessions

The duration of the sessions is, in general, forty-five minutes, which allows the patients to settle into therapeutic time and to take up life on the psychosomatic level. In some cases, the time of the sessions can be reduced to thirty minutes if the patient has real difficulties, often of a narcissistic nature, in settling down during the sessions; it will then be a question of establishing the acceptance of a certain passivity to allow difficult emotional events to be relived in the session.

In psychoanalysis in the strict sense, missed sessions are paid for and the patient must adapt to the psychoanalyst's holiday dates. I am referring here to the practices of the classical psychoanalysts of the International Association of Psychoanalysis.

What, then, about psychosomatic therapies? I recommend flexibility: my practice is to ask the patient either to notify me one week in advance of his absence, telling him that I will be able to devote the time of his session to another patient, so that that he appreciates my professional practice; or warn me two days before the session; or I adapt to the patient who is very fragile, offering him the opportunity to warn me even later.

We must adapt to the patient according to the diagnosis and the fragility of his defences (serious illnesses, hospitalisations, etc.). As for holidays, the patient is free to take them when he wishes. Once this practice is stated, any missed session is down to the patient, which allows us to understand the missed act. If the patient has a serious illness, we can introduce more flexibility, and move the session to another day or time of the week. Let's not forget that we have patients with serious illnesses, that they are often undergoing very heavy chemotherapy and that they need to recover. We must take this into account; it is not forbidden to visit them in the hospital. If the patient is not present in the first fifteen minutes of the session, I am like a worried mother and I will call him on his mobile.

I am flexible enough around these criteria because we are always facing a severe superego or facing an implacable ego ideal. It is also important in the case of psychosomatist training seminars that I do not become for my colleagues an institutional superego that will disrupt their professional functioning. What should be done? I recommend a certain direction for the therapeutic process and it is up to the future psychosomatists, if they do not agree, to find the most favourable way to practice provided that the course of the cure can always be understood. Quite often, during some of my courses in the training of therapists, I find that they were completely conditioned by their initial training: future therapists must follow very strict rules. These are trainings where the institutional superego predominates, without explanation, which is quite harmful to the psychic functioning and autonomy of future psychotherapists.

Follow-up

The essential goal to pursue is the health of our patients. Let's not forget that somatic patients can see their symptoms worsen between sessions or their symptoms regress and it is essential we understand developments. I remember that the first time I was confronted with the problematic of somatic patients, it was more than thirty-five years ago, within the framework of the Society of Psychoanalysis. A psychoanalyst was talking about a cancer patient he had lost, and he described how he had had this patient lie down. It must be understood that, cut off from the therapist's perception and sensory mechanics, the patient can regress very quickly and become disorganised somatically, feeling abandoned. It is always important, as I have often taught, to assess psychosomatic risk; one cannot ask a patient suffering from a serious illness to lie down.

We psychosomaticists must accompany and control the regressive movements of our patients. If you want a patient to lie down, it is best to move the chair to face the couch so that the patient can see you. You combine a regressive movement while remaining in the patient's line of sight. All patients with significant sensorimotor fixation and early-life deficiencies who are starting to talk about drug dependence pathologies or immune system depression should be confronted face to face because being able to see us is fundamental. When there is a mental recovery, we can gradually move from a maternal attachment relationship and gradually switch to an oedipal triangulation with the appearance of the father. We move from an archaic and pregenital model of functioning to an oedipal model of functioning. This was the case with my patient who, after two months of regression and recovery of new psychosomatic balances, wrote to me to tell me that she had organised and programmed her weekend, something she had never done before since she had spent all her weekends "breaking down". A paternal transfer began to take place, and I think that in the coming months an oedipal triangulation will appear. The energy modification develops gradually as she invests in movement: gym, walks in the forest, arranging her apartment.

In severe cases, it is advisable to accompany the therapy with a medical follow-up, namely to make contact, with the agreement of the patient, with the attending physician to inquire about the evolution of the somatic symptoms. When patients are going to be operated on, I advise going with them to the hospital or clinic where they are to have the operation. They need to know that you are there as a sort of maternal protective authority that does not abandon them. We can have very warm contact with our hospitalised patients and even hold their hand if that is desirable and comforting. I remember a cancer patient I consulted at the hospital who jumped into my arms at the end of the session to give me a kiss. We must understand the nature of the emotional relationships that develop between our patients and ourselves; this cancer patient, who is still in therapy with me, regularly gives me chocolates on New Year's Day. I know that there are prohibitions of a psychoanalytic nature on physical touch with our patients, for fear of an eroticisation of the relationship. I understand these warnings very well, and it's up to you to make sure you implement what we call the abstinence rule. That should not stop you from being, as Winnicott says, "a good enough mother".

You must understand the different stages that a human being goes through to become an adult; it is a difficult path that reactivates our own journey with consequences on our countertransference. If the notion of mentalization needs to be specified, we must question the myth of the very good mentalization that protects diseases! At the Pierre Marty Institute of Psychosomatics, we developed the belief that mental wellbeing was immune to disease. My practice over twenty years and many psychosomatic epidemiological studies have demonstrated quite the opposite, validating the statement of Joyce McDougall that "no one is safe from somatisations".

About the imaginary and the preconscious

Using the psychosomatic risk assessment method, we can establish a diagnosis evaluating the breadth of the preconscious, that is to say, the extent of the importance of its imaginary necessary for mental elaboration with associative capacities, the solidity of the links between the present and the past; we can also evaluate the strength of the links between the evocation of a life event and its relationship with emotions. It is obvious that if a patient does not fulfil the minimum organisational conditions of the first Freudian topic, the associative capacities will be limited and it is recommended then to resort to psycho-corporal therapies to restore the image of the body and, in the long run, the associative capacities of the patient.

There are also patients who are in an eternal present, according to Joyce McDougall (1978) who describes them as normopaths and that Pierre Marty classified as neuroses of behaviour (see the cases discussed). You can also meet somatic patients who have enormous problems with the body, whose narcissistic pathology is in denial of the body. These patients think that they exist outside their body and, therefore, cannot follow medical prescriptions. In these cases, it is better to resort to a body-relaxation psychotherapist or the many orientations of body psychotherapy including, of course, the psycho-corporal therapies of traditional Chinese medicine. This type of therapy allows the gradual restoration of the psychic image of the body and thus ultimately of the continuity of psychosomatic unity.

Psychoanalysts speak of "psychosomatisation" of the body. We are in the presence of two images: a psychic image and a neurological image. Once the psychosomatic unit is re-established, the patients gain or regain an associative activity allowing the breadth of the preconscious to be reconstituted. After one or two years of body psychotherapy, the relaxation psychotherapist can refer you again to patients who have re-established their mental capacities. I am in no way opposed to the cognitive and behavioural therapies practised by my psychiatrist colleagues at Pitié-Salpêtrière because these techniques can contribute to the restoration of the continuity of the psychosomatic unit in the cognitive and corporal domains necessary to the restoration of the functioning of a psychic apparatus. I bear in mind that the psychic system interrelates behaviours, emotions, and mental representations (of things and words), so CBTs (cognitive and behavioural therapies) contribute to the development of the psychic system but are insufficient to restore overall functioning.

I am very open to all the techniques allowing the restoration of the continuity of the psychosomatic unit provided that these techniques are used in a way that is complementary to the psychosomatic therapies and facilitates their evolution. I am much attached to the re-establishment of the psychic system based on the interrelation between behaviours, emotions, and mental representations. In my hospital consultation, I sometimes received patients who had been treated with hypnosis (EMDR) and cognitive and behavioural therapies, and so on, who come to supplement their treatments because they realise they are not sufficient. Our main work is to restore overall balance of the psychic apparatus and, at the same time, the balance of the neural networks. Our job as a psychosomatist is to build links, to construct the huge psychic network that stretches from the most distant past to the present day.

The problem of the payment of the sessions

The payment can be made in cash, which is preferable since it is a test of the anal and narcissistic control of patients and is a reality test. The payment relationship is often surprising because the compulsion of repetition will show itself: forgetting the payment at the end of the session, or if the patient writes a cheque, errors in the amount or the spelling of the name of the therapist; these are manifestations of latent aggression that will allow us to reactivate in the patient many memories of past repressed conflict events. Patient–therapist conflicts will activate the whole relationship with the anality and aggressive control impulses of the other. It is important to be very comfortable with the manifestations of the anal drive since we live in a country where the ideological-cultural criticism of this impulse is dominant is (France, unlike the Anglo-Saxon countries, has a very significant oral culture; its cuisine is world famous). In other cultural universes, this impulse is accepted, as well as the pleasure related to this drive: for example, earning money without guilt.

The regularity of the payment is fundamental to the continuation of the treatment. You can request a payment at the end of each session or at the end of each month, at best. For somatic patients, it is preferable that the payment is made at the end of each session because the regularity of this payment will gradually ensure better pregenital control on the part of the patients who will integrate it into the process of psychosexual maturation.

Questions asked by the participants in the seminar at the Society of Integrative Psychosomatics

With regard to the role of the mother

If at diagnosis, maternal deprivation and lack of introjection of the maternal image are found, then it is up to you to fulfil this role in the attachment relationship, which may take between nine and eighteen months to be introjected. It is obvious that such an exercise requires, especially for male therapists, much of the feminine side of your psyche. It is also important that you have theoretical models of metapsychology and integrative psychosomatics that help you to restore the mental representations of patients. Often, I imagine that I am in front of a huge tapestry that I must repair; I also imagine that I am exploring an immense building and that sometimes I must go down, that is to say, regress, into the basement and not stay in the upper floors because there I will be unable to communicate with my patient.

Interventions are intended to prepare, repair, or to build the psychic apparatus. We are in a situation that is very different from that in psychoanalysis, since we are dealing with significant shortcomings of preconsciousness.

Whole periods disappear momentarily from conscious awareness through trauma, and our work is to help in the construction of the story of the patient: the "storytelling". The analysis of the defences by the lifting of the repression will allow the emergence of buried memories, reconstituting the frame of the life events. This reconstitution will, in certain cases, when the psychosomatic unit is restored, allow us to see the oedipal conflict come up.

Thus, in one of my books (Stora, 2013), I demonstrate the case of Damien, who consulted me at the hospital for hypochondriacal disorders, effectively masking colorectal cancer. The psychosomatic therapy of the first four years, combined with the medical treatments, restored the continuity of the psychosomatic unit. Then the oedipal conflict appeared and was analysed according to the classical technique of psychoanalysis before ending the treatment by mutual agreement, while the analysed oedipal organisation facilitated the reorganisation of the psychosomatic unit. We can often be very surprised at the re-establishment of psychosomatic unity; I have seen, in the case of transplant patients, a revival of the desire for children, much to the chagrin of transplant surgeons. The messages sent by the body to the patients will activate the desires of children, thus disrupting the medical contraindications as well as the doctors who did not understand the consequences of the transplant reviving the life instinct. These patients will sometimes endanger the foetus during pregnancy and it is our duty to explain to doctors the psychic problem underlying them, that is, the consequences of their surgical work.

The restoration of somatic and libidinal energy balance will often allow the preconscious to restore its integrity and some neurotic symptoms to disappear, in the same way as we saw during the war, namely a temporary disappearance of neuroses. In breast cancer research, we can see in some patients that the energy mobilised by cancerous tumours re-establishes or, rather, establishes, a new psychic equilibrium, giving a new meaning to life. The ways in which psychosexual energy is redirected by the disease lead patients to view their lives and their environment in a different way. The defence systems of somatic patients are often very archaic and we are in the presence of what Freud calls a "return to oneself", that is to say, a breaking down of the instincts or rather an instinctual non-entanglement of the aggressive impulses. Aggressive drives turn against the self and attack it, as if to bring about self-destruction. We must then gradually remove the inhibition of the aggressive impulses so that the ego can reinvest the object which will allow a reintroduction of the drive.

With regard to the fundamental danger

In my opinion, we must discuss all the problems around the possibility of putting our somatic patients' lives in danger; for the moment I prefer to declare that it is important to protect the lives and psychic balance of the children of our patients. This is an absolute duty, and practically the only intervention we need to make beyond those regarding the dangers of our patients' suicides. We must not underestimate the role of somatic pathologies, which may worsen during treatment or be interpreted as resistance to psychotherapy.

During the psychosomatic interview, we know for certain that the patient will not reveal all the information concerning his illness, let alone his psychic functioning; what remains hidden will represent all the work we have to do in psychosomatic psychotherapy. In addition, we are often faced with two different presentations: the illness as narrated by the patient and the illness as established by the doctor during the clinical examination.

Here are a few tips and recommendations that it is up to future psychosomaticists to take up; after having read them, they will be able to follow their own path. It is essential that the future psychosomatist has freedom of choice in their practice.

From the psychoanalytic clinic to psychosomatic therapy: the role of the analytic cure in the training of the integrative psychosomatic psychotherapist

The practice of psychosomatic psychotherapies implies that the psychosomatic psychotherapist has first performed work on himself by resorting to the technique known as the classic psychoanalytic treatment. Without knowledge of his unconscious, it is difficult for the psychosomatic psychotherapist, whether he be a doctor or a therapist, to undertake treatment of somatic patients. The so-called classical cure is the model from which all other psychotherapeutic treatments have evolved over the last one hundred years.

I began to practice psychoanalysis in 1973, and since then I have continued my self-analysis and to question myself about my own psychoanalysis carried out within the psychoanalytic society of the International Psychoanalytical Association (IPA). The model developed by Freud and adopted by the members of the IPA began to seem incomplete; for example, cultural differences seemed to be absent from the analytical process as it is practiced in France. And, as it appeared much later, in the late 1980s and thanks to Joyce McDougall's contributions, the problems of identity, and how they were constituted, were totally absent from the analytic process. Also absent were the affects and their manifestation, the experience of present and past situations, as well as the in-depth understanding of psychodynamic conflict. The behaviour of psychoanalysts vis-à-vis their patients was also the subject of questioning on my part. Why this intellectual approach? Why this pseudo-distance and this apparent coldness?

At this point, I think it is time to question the history of the establishment of the model of the classic cure to understand how this model differed from the approach developed by Sándor Ferenczi, who, along with Melanie Klein, inspired the practice of psychosomatic therapy. I knew Ferenczi, thanks to my relations with the colleagues of the Hungarian Society of Psychoanalysis.[31] In France, in the 1970s, at the Institute of Psychoanalysis, Ferenczi was never spoken about, but I never questioned this; given my North African origins, where respect for teachers is at the heart of the relationship, I held in high esteem, and deeply respected, the teaching I received without ever questioning those who dispensed it. I had to go through many stages before I could put everything in perspective, so that our association[32] can benefit from the lessons of the past, and we can embark on a different path where tolerance must guide our scientific and professional relations.

It all began in the 1920s, a crucial time for the future of the IPA. The problem was first raised within the students' committee and amongst the disciples of Freud, with important consequences for the practice of contemporary psychoanalysis, which favours the classical oedipal genital cure. In presenting his model, Freud stayed with his model of 1916 with regard to transference, and, in 1938, in his overview of psychoanalysis, he remains attached to a work of construction work carried out in collaboration with the patient driven by the power of the transference. He continues to focus the cure on remembering, by looking for confirmation of the experience, whether it be traumatic or simply fantasy, and seeking out the oedipal core of the repressed events while attempting to reconstruct the patient's story.

---

[31] These relationships have been established with the help of my French-speaking wife, Professor Judith Stora-Sándor, professor emeritus at the University of Paris 8.

[32] Excerpt from a lecture delivered to the Society of Interactive Psychosomatics.

Since 1910, he had been emphasising the importance of the psycho-analyst's emotional dimension (the problem of countertransference), without making it part of the therapeutic relationship, and in 1912 he introduced the need for a personal analysis as a prerequisite for professional practice. Remember that it was only from 1925 that what is called didactic analysis was developed. As for the transference, Freud remained in the position of the father because the position of the mother embarrassed him significantly. He developed the notion of free-floating attention, that is, free from any act of coming to a conclusion or of bringing things together, devoid of any personal interference on the part of the analyst or any presuppositions about what he might hear or discover. But in his practice, Freud was very different: he spoke to his patients in a friendly way, he helped patients in financial difficulties, he accepted gifts, he invited his patients to dine with his family, he analysed his own daughter Anna, etc. (Jones, 1953).

In truth, this was a practice far removed from theoretical statements and recommendations! The transference, the compulsion to repeat, the revealing of meaning to patients, the awareness—all this proves to be insufficient to produce psychic change. Freud does not modify his technique; he is tired of this therapeutic process of the cure he has established; he prefers theoretic investigation and it is this that he privileges in his practice.

Reshaping the setting of the cure

From 1921, Freud's notoriety attracted many patients for whom he could not guarantee a treatment; he preferred to refer them to Sándor Ferenczi, who was his friend and his number two in the psychoanalytic institution. At this point, he reorganised the setting of the cure: from six weekly sessions to five so that other patients can be accepted; this practice would be built into the canonical rules of the cure later on. The analyses were shortened, lasting only a few months and the conditions set up in advance, along with the duration of the treatment, the fee, price increases ... A patient of Freud describes the course of psychoanalysis thus: locate the Oedipus complex, interpret repressed homosexuality, and, from there, allow the patient to do the rest, namely work everything through.

During the 1920s, one thinks of the psychoanalytic training analysis which is regarded favourably by Sigmund Freud. In this period, he devoted his time to the study of culture, religion, civilisation, and applying psychoanalysis to other disciplines: *Civilisation and its Discontents, Moses and Monotheism*, etc. This was an extraordinary time, when new psychoanalytic approaches were born: Sándor Ferenczi, through his analytical practice, met somatic patients, and he understood that the oedipal genital model did not apply! He began to develop critical propositions describing another approach to the treatment of patients. In 1910 he had become the first President of the IPA and still held the position. He had begun to suffer from Biermer's anaemia (pernicious anaemia), of which he died in 1933. Ferenczi informed Freud, by letter, about his health problems, Freud repeatedly told him that this was a "flight into illness". Later, he wrote that he did not believe Ferenczi was organically ill. Here again, we can see the first psychoanalyst's approach to truly organic disorders; he does not recognise their importance or the consequences for the health of the patient.

I want to point out here, and warn you against, some psychoanalytic beliefs about organic disease; even hypochondria (cf. the case of one of my hypochondriacal cases, Stora, 2013) can mask a serious illness. We must always be very careful. In 1924, Sándor Ferenczi and Otto Rank, in *The Development of Psychoanalysis* (1984), anticipated a clinic that emphasises feelings and the lived experience. These proposals were opposed to those of Freud, creating a climate of hostility in which they were rejected; they were unacceptable and remain unacceptable for orthodox psychoanalytic societies. I recall that in the British Psychoanalytical Society, there were three groups: Kleinians, Anna Freudians, and the Middle Group.

It is obvious that the conception of the cure as discussed above is less comfortable for the psychoanalyst since he exposes his person and the countertransference is present in the relationship. For Ferenczi, it was important that analysis does not become an end in itself. Freud initially adopted an ambivalent attitude, and then ended up criticising the positions of Rank and Ferenczi, which opened the door to violent criticism of their followers. Their work was blacklisted and their names condemned to oblivion, at least in the IPA. Psychoanalytic ideology took precedence over the scientific approach.

In the history of the analytic movement, preference is given to the preservation of Sigmund Freud's invention, as if it were threatened! Ferenczi and Rank warned against too much intellectualisation, against the risk that the cure would become an end in itself; they advocated giving a significant place to affect. Ferenczi wanted to take care of the patient, and persisted in trying to improve his method; he was never satisfied with theoretical certainties, which was, in a way, a violation of the purity of Freud's invention. It is possible that Freud struggled with Ferenczi's criticism: with the element of rivalry and with the narcissistic attacks on the cure.

The year 1924 was one of very violent reactions against Ferenczi and Rank; *The Development of Psychoanalysis* was dismantled, to be published in France seventy years later! Otto Rank was excluded from the psychoanalytic movement. Recall that in his book *The Trauma of Birth*, Otto Rank (1929) develops the idea that the first biological separation from the mother can constitute the prototype of anxiety. It is therefore in this mode of maternal and pre-oedipal transference that the relationship of the patient to the analyst can be interpreted within the treatment. He sees in the attachment to the mother a possible interpretation that will shorten the time needed for the cure. Psychoanalysts criticised the maternal transference by identifying it with the transference to the archaic mother, thus denouncing the transference that harms the patient by causing him to regress instead of engaging him in a progressive movement. This was the opinion, and may still be the opinion, of the psychoanalysts in the member societies of the IPA. As you know, in the context of the psychosomatic integrative psychosomatic psychotherapy that I advocate and propose, given the pregenital and archaic problems of many somatic patients, we must play the role of the mother: not the archaic mother, but the genital mother who takes care of and repairs the narcissistic integrity of the disease that has caused the regressions of which we are aware. There is no question of remaining at the regressive stage achieved by our patients; on the contrary, we should enable them to progress to reach a durable equilibrium compatible with an improvement in their health.

Otto Rank and Sándor Ferenczi say that we must encourage in the patient the tendency to reproduce, in the treatment, old situations and forgotten infantile emotions; to allow feelings of abandonment, love, hatred, jealousy towards the therapist, in the knowledge that these are only transpositions of feelings experienced in childhood with regard to parental figures. It is a question of encouraging their emergence so as to transform them, for the patient, into current memories. The activity of the therapist is neither injunction nor total prohibition; it is based on the ability of the psychoanalyst to fulfil the role prescribed to him by the patient's unconscious. By relieving early traumatic experiences, the patient can experience an awareness that is not only given to him by the analyst but that he has already experienced and felt.

For these two authors:

> Analyses have been conducted up to this point in a way that is too intellectual, which is why they often shows limitations, and why they often drag on. Analysts insist very strongly on living, in the cure, this experience of the past; these analysts have many patients who have understood their treatment, and their own psychic functioning, intellectually, continue to behave in a neurotic way. To overinterpret, that is, to prove to the patient that he has complexes, would have no other effect than to reduce psychoanalysis to an intellectual approach. We must live the affects in the present and not be limited to an explanatory process of past affect.
>
> (Millet, 2010)

In conclusion, for Sándor Ferenczi, therapeutic analyses have become, more and more, didactic analyses aiming at transmitting the theory elaborated by Freud rather than developing the patient's psychoanalytical process.

The psychoanalysis of the orthodox schools oppose birth trauma and, thus, the archaic maternal relationship to the Oedipus complex. This opposition, these quarrels, the side-lining of Sándor Ferenczi and Otto Rank, reveal today a lack of understanding of the process of psychosexual maturation, and of the metapsychological model. As I have pointed out throughout this book, there is a continuum, from birth to the end of this process, which integrates the psychic dimension and the neuronal dimension (see Stora, 2011).

The cure must follow the progress of this process and facilitate its recovery. What about the oedipal genital issue? It varies with each patient. In some cases, we can stabilise the process at a pregenital stage of development that allows patients to continue their lives by leaving "our door open" to either support patients or continue their analyses. We can thus arrive at the genital stage and continue our treatments, according to the procedures of the so-called classic cure. The arrival at the genital stage is often spectacular: at the end of the illness, the psychosomatic unit is reconstituted, and the life drive revives the process of maturation which resumes its forward progress.

Given the fragility of somatic patients, and their archaic and pregenital fixations, the attitude of the psychosomatist is, first, to take a maternal role to help the development of the psychic system and the smooth process of maturation to unlock the fixation points and then, in the best cases, to tackle the oedipal conflict. It must be understood, however, that this is not so for all patients.

Before concluding, I wish to pay tribute to Sándor Ferenczi and briefly return to the conflicts created by his new approach to patients. In fact, we found ourselves, in the 1920s, at a strategic and dramatic crossroads of theory and practice, especially in terms of how the practice of psychoanalysis was conceived. While the French societies of the IPA still, nowadays, exist in a narrow orthodoxy of Freudian practice, it was not true of the British Psychoanalytical Society, which, by accepting the coexistence of many different currents of practice, never excluded the partisans of Ferenczi's clinic.

We owe this to the Hungarian School of Psychoanalysis of which Sándor Ferenczi was the leader, having influenced his students and disciples: Melanie Klein, Michael Balint, his friends and colleagues Geza Roheim, Franz Alexander, etc.[33] These analysts strongly influenced the next generation, of which Winnicott was a remarkable example. We know that all these great contemporary analysts (with Winnicott in the foreground) consider the affects and the importance of interpreting,

---

[33] I will add to these analysts, Wilfred Bion, Daniel Stern, and Françoise Dolto.

in the framework of the analytic relationship, the determining role played by the countertransference of the psychoanalyst. I, myself, have long advocated psychosomatic therapies by emphasising the same dimensions. Whatever the criticism of Sándor Ferenczi, his pioneering attempts paved the way for what I now call integrative psychosomatic psychotherapy.

For the Society of Integrative Psychosomatics, I wish for an attitude based on tolerance, the exclusion of ideology contrary to the scientific spirit, and a discussion about practices to better treat our patients by considering the evolution of our contemporary cultures and societies. We must move resolutely forward into the future by insisting on a spirit of tolerance and openness.

Appendix 1

Notes on the following form:

First, I would like to thank, very warmly, Dr Lionel Naccache who suggested to me to modify the statistical procedure of adding the scores of the different dimensions of the psychosomatic unit. Such an addition, in truth, is irrelevant to the extent that the subjective scores led the psychosomatic observer (born) to weight each of the dimensions which is an absolute error. It is important, with the modifications made, to take into account the overall picture and to compare with the knowledge we have today, the scores of the different dimensions to arrive at an unquantified qualitative observation of the overall psychosomatic risk. For epidemiological studies, it will be easier to establish cross-tabulations by retaining each of the dimensions of the psychosomatic unit crossed for each disease with the biological variables communicated by the medical profession. The somatic risk should be identified using the usual biological variables.

Second, it is important to note that a first classification was developed by Pierre Marty (1987). My method, which is not a classification, takes into consideration the work of Pierre Marty and is profoundly modified by the approach of integrative psychosomatics. I took up the concepts of psychoanalysis developed by Sigmund Freud and those who came after him, to which I added all my research on occupational stress and induced somatic disorders.

RESULTS OF THE PSYCHOSOMATIC CLINICAL EXAMINATION

Method to facilitate the establishment of the risk of the psychosomatic unit in its six dimensions

JBS-PSYSOMA: version 25 April 2020
Developed by J. B. STORA from 1993 to 2021

PATIENT RECORD

Last name: ——————————— First name: ———————————

Date of birth: ————————————

Start date of treatment: ————————————

End of treatment date: ————————————

History of the disease: information collected in the medical record, see Axis 5 of the grid.

Please use the International Classification of Diseases.

History of the patient: grid to be completed after investigation.

Overall assessment of psychosomatic functioning: with determination of the risk profile. To be completed only after establishing the patient's history, psychic functioning, and somatic disorders.

The summary table is at the end of the grid and must be completed after filling in the headings.

This grid must be completed at the beginning, during, and at the end of processing:

Diagnosis, prognosis, therapeutic strategy.

Summary table of life events and somatic disorders with comments
Your comments should help you to gradually establish the characteristics of psychic functioning (behaviour, thoughts, emotions, mental representations) by replacing them in the patient's family and professional environment in order to establish a first diagnosis. After following the patient for six months you can review the initial diagnosis and consider the therapeutic strategy.

Feedback	Life events	Dates or ages	Somatic disorders
Feedback	Life events	Dates or ages	Somatic disorders

PATIENT RECORD

Last name: _________________________   First name: _________________________

Date of birth: _________________________

Date of clinical examination: _________________________

Recommendation: Once you have assigned a score to each of the dimensions of the psychosomatic unit, group them into the summary table at the end of the examination of the six dimensions. This table will allow you to establish a diagnosis, a prognosis, and a direction for the cure.

1. **Processes and psychic mechanisms**	1. Trauma during the mother's pregnancy. 1a. Trauma and maternal deficiency during the first year of life. 1b. Family obstacles to the development of the psychic system; hindrance to the development of infantile neurosis, predominance of motor behaviours. Fragility of the Self. 1c. Absence of internalisation of the Object, non-entanglement of impulses, reversal of aggressive impulses against Self, self-destruction, aggravation of somatisations and traumas; predominant attachment relationship. 2. Functioning of the balanced psychic system: ability to remember the past; ability to go back and forth between the present and the past; ability to develop mentally.	Note: Psychic functioning

<ul><li>**Axis 1A:** object relationship:<ul><li>1: presence of the object</li><li>2: evaluation of the narcissistic dimension (grandiose Self presence, ideal of the Self)</li><li>3: the masochistic dimension</li><li>4: the thickness of the pre-conscious (imagination, associations, dreams)</li></ul></li><li>**Axis 1B:** psychic states and personal life events:<ul><li>anxieties</li><li>bereavement</li><li>depression</li><li>trauma</li><li>influence of culture</li></ul></li><li>**Axis 1C:** somatic fixations<ul><li>psychic fixations</li></ul></li></ul>	3. Momentarily impaired psychic functioning: Irregularities of mental functioning—momentary overflows of the possibilities of mental elaboration by excess of excitement or repression of representations. 4. Impaired psychic functioning: life and operative thinking. 5. Severely impaired psychic functioning: progressive disorganisations (essential depression). Assessment of the risk related to the functioning and dysfunctions of the psychic system *stricto sensu.*	
	Absence of constant risk, temporary overflow: Moderate to high risk:<ul><li>possibility of reversibility, reorganisation from the points of fixation-regression, monitoring, instability.</li></ul>High to very high risk:<ul><li>overall instability of the psychic dimension of the disorganised psychosomatic unit.</li></ul>	

• **Axis 1D:** defence mechanisms
• **Axis 1E:** presence of character traits:
  • phobic
  • hysterical
  • perverse
  • predominantly oral
  • predominantly anal
  • phallic-narcissistic
  • sado-masochistic relationship
	Therapeutic indications:
	• High-risk subject— overall instability of the disorganised psychosomatic unit.
	• Medium-risk subject— possibility of reversibility of symptoms, reorganisation from fixation points. Monitor for possible instability.
	• Low-risk subject, high potential for reorganisation.
	• Stable subject affected by a temporary overflow of the psychic apparatus.	

2. Economic resources (libidinal energy and somatic energy)		
Resources: Axis 1F: assess the resources usually available to the patient when he or she faces life's difficulties: **Grade from Level 1 to Level 4 (low, medium, high, very high):** • spiritual resources • dream resources • writing activities • sports activities It should be understood that it is a question of evaluating the energy balance (the principle of economy) because the disease can absorb a very large amount of somatic energy to heal itself. This is the self-repair of the psychosomatic unit and the energy mobilised by the somatic defences.		Note: Resources

3. Prevalence of behaviours: 1. controlled and integrated behaviour 2. low 3. average 4. strong		
4. Capacity for the expression of affects: 1. well-integrated representations and affects 2. repression with three possible outcomes (displacement ex phobia, obsessions; loosened from representation: ex hysteria; transformation; ex neurosis anxiety) 3. predominance of vitality affects in the relationship 4. affects representing the memory of a traumatic unrepresentable experience 5. alexithymia		

5. Somatic risk The body, organs, and functions; the biological parameters of reference of doctors.		Four levels: Based on observation results, diagnosis, and prognosis communicated by the patient's doctors: • very high risk • high risk • medium risk • low risk
6. Environmental risk Nature of the environment (family environment and professional environment). The examination assesses the adaptability implemented and/or the possible harms to psychosomatic health (trauma): 1. very satisfactory level 2. satisfactory 3. slight temporary alteration 4. difficulties of medium intensity 5. significant alteration 6. major impairment leading to temporary incapacity for functioning 7. long-term inability to function independently		Environment family and professional environment. The examination assesses the adaptability implemented and/or the possible harms to psychosomatic health (trauma).

Diagnosis according to benign psychosomatic nosography

<table>
<tr><td colspan="6">Overall assessment of psychosomatic functioning
Diagnosis and therapeutic strategy</td></tr>
<tr><td colspan="6">You must compare in the table below the six dimensions of the psychosomatic unit in order to arrive at the assessment of the overall psychosomatic risk according to systems theory (JBS). The addition of scores is irrelevant.</td></tr>
<tr><td>Psyche</td><td>Resources</td><td>Comportment</td><td>Effects</td><td>Soma</td><td>Environment</td></tr>
<tr><td></td><td></td><td></td><td></td><td></td><td></td></tr>
<tr><td></td><td></td><td></td><td></td><td></td><td></td></tr>
<tr><td></td><td></td><td></td><td></td><td></td><td></td></tr>
</table>

You must give your conclusions (diagnosis and prognosis) above, e.g. high vulnerability, difficulties in observing treatments, recommendation for psychotherapeutic follow-up, etc. Doctors need to have conclusions to better appreciate the evolution of their patients.

Signature of the psychosomatic psychotherapist

____

Appendix 2

Dynamic psychosomatic nosograpy
Established on 19/11/2008 by Jean Benjamin Stora

Once the psychic functioning, and the reactions to the environment, have been established you can then propose a diagnosis from the table below.

The psychosomatic diagnosis is established from the four dimensions of psychic functioning and the patient's relationship to the environment; it is thus possible to propose an assessment of the psychosomatic risk by integrating the somatic risk communicated by the doctors (see above). These descriptors will allow you to place the patient in the following three categories:

1. transfer neuroses, classical neuroses in the sense of psychoanalytic indications
2. current neuroses
3. Self-preserving, non-neurotic axis: narcissistic disorders of the Self, identity, and behaviour (original insufficiency of the preconscious—disorganisation)
4. psychoses (for psychoses and mood disorders, we advise you to refer to the DSM-IV manual)

The psychosomatic functional structures below are dynamic and not immovable

Nosographic classification	Diagnostic
1. Transfer neuroses (defence psychoneuroses (S. Freud)) (well-mentalized neurosis: certainty)	
	Obsessive neurosis
Symptoms	Phobia
	Hysteria
Symptomatically organised mental neurosis, with sustained functioning	Polymorphic neuroses without dominant and sustained mental symptomatology These may be organisations with transient obsessive manifestations or hysterical organisations with phenomena of conversion; neurotic or psychotic mental systematics have been overwhelmed by conflict, at least momentarily (P. Marty, 1987)
Prevalence of conversion symptoms	Conversion hysteria
Symptom: phobia	Anxiety hysteria (term created by S. Freud)
2. Current neuroses Failure of the constitution of infantile neurosis Neurosis with uncertain mentalization: doubt Poorly mentalized neurosis: proven defects Mentalization suddenly appreciates three fundamental qualities of the preconscious: thickness of all the representative formations; fluidity of the links between the representations; usual permanence of the functioning	
	Neurosis of anxiety
	Neurosis of character
	Hypochondria (different states)
	Traumatic neurosis
	Neurosis of the relationship to the allergic object

<table>
<tr><td colspan="2">3. Self-preservative axis
Narcissistic disorders of the Self, identity, and behaviour
(original insufficiency of the preconscious—non-mentalized
inorganisation-neuroses)</td></tr>
<tr><td></td><td>Neurosis of behaviour</td></tr>
<tr><td></td><td>Archaic hypochondria</td></tr>
<tr><td></td><td>Narcissism disorders</td></tr>
<tr><td></td><td>Identity disorders</td></tr>
<tr><td></td><td>Troubles addictifs</td></tr>
<tr><td></td><td>"Cold psychosis" or non-delusional (A. Green., E. Kestemberg)</td></tr>
<tr><td colspan="2">4. Delusional psychoses
Consult the DSM-IV diagnostic method for all psychoses and mood disorders</td></tr>
<tr><td colspan="2">Schizophrenia and other psychotic disorders</td></tr>
<tr><td colspan="2">Mood disorders</td></tr>
<tr><td colspan="2">Anxiety disorders</td></tr>
<tr><td colspan="2">Dissociative difficulties</td></tr>
<tr><td colspan="2">Gender-identity disorders</td></tr>
<tr><td colspan="2">Eating disorders</td></tr>
<tr><td>Adjustment disorders</td><td>With depressed mood, with anxiety, with disruption of behaviors, with disruption of both emotions and non-specific behaviours</td></tr>
<tr><td>Personality disorders</td><td>Paranoid, schizoid, antisocial, borderline, histrionic, narcissistic, avoidant, dependent, obsessive-compulsive, non-specific</td></tr>
<tr><td colspan="2">Refer to the DSM-IV manual for more details</td></tr>
</table>

Appendix 3

Behavioural neurosis

In his book *Les Mouvements individuels de vie et de mort: Essai d'économie psychosomatique* (*The Individual Movements of Life and Death: An Essay in Psychosomatic Economics*), Pierre Marty addresses the problem of neurotic behaviour whose vital tone is uncertainty. Behavioural neuroses include many basic vital organisations: a combination of short, more or less evolved organisational paths with sublimations, perversions, neurotic, or psychotic traits. This is the absence of the central chain of fixations with a deficiency in the lateral evolutionary line.

> Note JBS: Pierre Marty refers here to the process of psychosexual maturation that takes place over time and constitutes what is called the central fixation chain; fixation since the point of development can stop at one of the stages of this process. What Marty calls the lateral evolutionary line is a development parallel to the process leading to genitality. As I write, no one is using this concept anymore. It is not operational at all. Only the concept of a central chain is still relevant.

The functional fragmentation of these structures is revealed in the movements of the relationship to the Other, in aspects of character and behaviour that are very disparate and especially unstable.

On the mental plane, the functioning of the first topic is poorly assured revealing the weakness of the preconscious constitution. At the level of the second topic, the oedipal superego is not constituted normally; by consequence we meet a self-ideal markedly little-developed from the all-powerful infant.

> Note JBS: Pierre Marty here advances a theoretical point that is in contradiction with the theoretical approach of psychosomatic integrative that I develop. Why? This is because we cannot talk about an oedipal superego if the process of psychosexual maturation has stopped upstream, by which I mean, at the archaic stage or the pregenital stage. In many cases, there is a complete lack of development of the transfer neurosis from the age of five or six. Therefore, to speak of the oedipal superego is a theoretical error.

In neuroses of behaviour, intrapsychic conflict does not exist in the psychoanalytic sense. It is rather a conflict with external objects equally invested in by the subject. Anxiety is lacking in the neurosis of behaviour, as is the feeling of guilt of the oedipal unconscious. Due to the functional insufficiency of the first topic, there is no fantasy activity, and mental elaboration is not possible. However, despite the subject's phantasmal poverty, communicable symbolic values remain: sublimated activities or works of art, for example. In these subjects, the attachment to the past as an ability to project themselves into the future is considerably diminished. The factual and the actual evidence of an operative life is already noticeable in the neurosis of behaviour. The difficulty of having a deep relationship with one's subjects is obvious, although the relationship can be very attractive when they express their interests or problems.

In these subjects, there are processes of secondary appearance in the form of intellectual or technical knowledge that may be confusing to the observer. Behaviours appear directly from the unconscious; sensorimotor functions constitute the elective way of expressing neurosis of behaviour. The interests of behavioural neurotics are directly attached to these functions. We can say that they remained fixed or attached to these functions.

> Note JBS: Advancing the sensorimotor dimension of neurotic behavioural patients very clearly indicates an archaic fixation with the hypothesis of an important maternal deficiency. The predominance of sensorimotor functions in behaviour reveals the immaturity of these patients.

We must differentiate between behaviour neurosis and acting out: in the acting out, the repression of the underlying fantasies implies a preconscious functioning with the possibility of subsequent emergence of these fantasies, which is not the case for behavioural neuroses. The same is true of lapses, forgetfulness, and missed acts. What must be noted is the presence of an unconscious that has not been enriched secondarily, with no other reference than that of immediate and incontestable reality. The notion of distance within the object, as found in mental neuroses, does not exist; we only meet the appreciation of real external distance, metric or geographical. This characteristic is close to or identical to that of the allergic object relation.

> Note JBS: there is, in fact, no preconscious instance since the imaginary of these patients is very poor, if not non-existent. All the contribution of the preconscious is to be made in the context of a therapeutic relationship. The fact that Pierre Marty evokes the distance to the object implies first that this object has not been internalised, which means that the distance to the object could not be constructed.

References

Anzieu, D. (1989). *The Skin Ego* (translated by C. Turner). New Haven, CT: Yale University Press.

Bion, W. R. (1961). A theory of thinking. *International Journal of Psychoanalysis, 43*, 306–310.

Bonaparte, M. (1958). Epilepsy and sadomasochism in the life and work of Dostoevsky. *French Review of Psychoanalysis, XXVI*(6).

Boston Change Process Study Group (2002). Explicating the implicit: The interactive microprocess in the analytic situation. *International Journal of Psychoanalysis, 83*, Report No. 3, 1051–1063.

Boston Change Process Study Group (2004). The something more than interpretation: Sloppiness and co-construction in the psychoanalytic encounter. *International Journal of Psychoanalysis, 85*, Report No. 4.

Bowlby, J. (1969). *Attachment and Loss, Vol. 1: Attachment.* London: Hogarth.

Checkland, P. (1981). *Systems Thinking, Systems Practice.* Chichester: John Wiley & Sons.

Damasio, A. R. (1999). *Le Sentiment même de soi. Corps, émotion, conscience* [*The Feeling of What Happens: Body and Emotion in the Making of Consciousness.* London: Vintage, 2000.]. Paris: Odile Jacob.

de Viel, E. (2010). Columnin. *Quotidien du Médecin*, 21 September.

Eaker, E. D., Abbott, R. D., & Kannell, W. B. (1989). Frequency of uncomplicated angina pectoris in type A compared with type B persons (the Framingham study). *American Journal of Cardiology, 63*(15): 1042–1045.

Fatorusso, V., & Rittter, O. (2006). *Vademecum clinique. Du diagnostic au traitement.* Paris: Masson.

Ferenczi S., & Rank O. (1984). *The Development of Psychoanalysis.* New York: International Universities Press. (*Perspective de la psychanalyse. Sur l'indépendance de la théorie et de la pratique.* Paris: Payot, 1924.)

Freud, S. (1893h). On the physical mechanism of hysterical phenomena: preliminary communication (with J. Breuer). *S. E. 2*: 1–18. London: Hogarth.

Freud, S. (1894). Draft E: How anxiety originates, 6 June 1894. In: J. M. Masson (Ed.), *The Complete Letters of Sigmund Freud to Wilhelm Fleiss, 1887–1904.* Cambridge, MA: Harvard University Press, 1985.

Freud, S. (1895b). On the grounds for detaching a particular syndrome from neurasthenia under the description "anxiety neurosis". *S. E., 3*: 87–120. London: Hogarth.

Freud, S. (1909b). Analysis of a phobia in a five-year-old boy. *S. E. 10*: 3–152. London: Hogarth.

Freud, S. (1912e). Recommendations to physicians practising psychoanalysis. *S. E. 12*: 109–156. London: Hogarth.

Freud, S. (1928d). Dostoevsky and parricide. *S. E. 21*: 177–194. London: Hogarth.

Freud, S. (1950a). Project for a scientific psychology. *S. E. 3*: 283–346. London: Hogarth.

Freud, S. (1961). *Letters of Sigmund Freud 1873–1939* (edited by E. L. Freud). London: Hogarth.

Friedman, M., Thoresen, C. E., Gill, J. J., Ulmer, D., Powell, L. H., Price, V. A., Brown, B., Thompson, L., Rabin, D. D., Breall, W. S., Bourg, E., Levy, R., & Dixon, T. (1986). Alteration of type A behaviour and its effects on cardiac recurrences in post myocardial infarction patients: Summary results of the recurrent coronary prevention project. *American Heart Journal, 112*: 653–665.

Green, A. (2009). *Resonance of Suffering: Countertransference in Non-neurotic Structures.* London: Karnac.

Grunberger, B. (2003). *Le Narcissisme* [*Narcissism: Psychoanalytic Essays.* New York: International Universities Press, 1991.]. Paris: Payot.

Jones, E. (1953). *The Life and Work of Sigmund Freud: Volume I*. New York: Basic Books.

Klein, M., Heimann, P., Isaacs, S., Rivière, J. (1966). *Développements de la psychanalyse* [*Developments in Psychoanalysis*. London: Hogarth, 1952.]. Paris: Presses Universitaires de France.

Kohut, H. (1971). *The Analysis of the Self: A Systematic Approach to the Psychoanalytic Treatment of Narcissistic Personality Disorders*. New York: International Universities Press.

Kübler-Ross, E. (1969). *On Death and Dying*. New York: Scribner.

Luria, A. R. (1972). *The Man With a Shattered World: The History of a Brain Wound* (translated by Lyn Solotaroff). Cambridge, MA: Harvard University Press. (*L'homme dont le monde volait en éclats* (translated by F. Mariengof & N. Rausch de Trautenberg). Paris: Seuil, 1995.)

Marty, P. (2006). La relation objectale allergique. *Revue française de psychanalyse, 22*(1): 30–35.

Merz, C. N., Krantz, D. S., & Rozanski, A. (1993). Mental stress and myocardial ischemia: Correlates and potential interventions. *Texas Heart Institute Journal, 20*: 152–157.

McDougall, J. (1978). *Plaidoyer pour une certaine abnormalité*. Paris: Gallimard. (*Plea for a Measure of Abnormality*. New York: Brunner/Mazel.)

McDougall, J. (1989). *Theaters of the Body*. New York: Norton.

Millet, A. (2010). *Psychanalystes, qu'avons-nous fait de la psychanalyse?* Paris: Seuil.

Naassila, M., & Pierrefiche, O. (2018). GluN2B Subunit of the NMDA receptor: The keystone of the effects of alcohol during neurodevelopment. *Neurochemical Research, 44*: 78–88.

Neyraut-Sutterman, M.-T. (2011). Parricide et épilepsie. À propos d'un article de Freud sur Dostoïevski. *Revue française de psychosomatique, 39*: 127–145.

Panksepp, J. (1998). *Affective Neuroscience: The Foundations of Human and Animal Emotions*. New York: Oxford University Press.

Rank, O. (1929). *The Trauma of Birth*. Abingdon, Oxon: Routledge.

Reich, P. (1983). How much does stress contribute to cardiovascular disease? *Journal of Cardiovascular Medicine, 8*: 825–831.

Rosenman, R. H., Brand, R. J., Sholtz, R. I., & Friedman, M. (1976). Multivariate prediction of coronary heart disease during 8.5 year follow-up in the Western Collaborative Group Study. *The American Journal of Cardiology, 37*(6), 903–910.

Schmidil, F. (1965). Freud and Dostoevsky. *Journal of the American Psychoanalytic Association*, *13*: 518–532.

Spitz, R. S. (1965). *The First Year of Life*. New York: International Universities Press.

Stora, J. B. (2007). *When the Body Displaces the Mind: Stress, Trauma and Somatic Disease* (preface by Mark Solms). London: Karnac.

Stora, J. B. (2011). *La neuropsychanalyse, controverses et dialogues* [*Neuropsychoanalysis, Controversies and Dialogues*]. Paris: MJW Fédition.

Stora, J. B. (2013). *La nouvelle approche psychosomatique. 9 cas cliniques* [*The New Psychosomatic Approach: 9 Clinical Cases*]. Paris: MJW Fédition.

Stora, J. B. (2018). The importance of psychic and neuronal factors in the evaluation of the somatic risk of breast cancer patients. *Journal of Integrative Psychosomatics*, *3*.

Strachey, J. (1934). The nature of the therapeutic action of psychoanalysis. *The International Journal of Psychoanalysis*, *15*: 127–159.

von Bertalanffy L. (1969). *General System Theory: Foundations, Development, Applications*. New York: George Braziller.

Winnicott, D. W. (1953). Transitional objects and transitional phenomena. *International Journal of Psychoanalysis*, *34*: 89–97.

Winnicott, D. W. (1967). Mirror-role of the mother and family in child development. In P. Lomas (Ed.), *The Predicament of the Family: A Psycho-Analytical Symposium* (pp. 26–33). London: Hogarth.

Winnicott, D. W. (1974). Fear of breakdown. *International Review of Psycho-Analysis*, *1*: 103–107.

Index